Gabriela Cavalcante da Silva
José Israel Guerra Junior

Drug Interactions and Prescription Profiles in Elderly Patients

Gabriela Cavalcante da Silva
José Israel Guerra Junior

Drug Interactions and Prescription Profiles in Elderly Patients

A Look at Pharmacotherapy

ScienciaScripts

Imprint

Any brand names and product names mentioned in this book are subject to trademark, brand or patent protection and are trademarks or registered trademarks of their respective holders. The use of brand names, product names, common names, trade names, product descriptions etc. even without a particular marking in this work is in no way to be construed to mean that such names may be regarded as unrestricted in respect of trademark and brand protection legislation and could thus be used by anyone.

Cover image: www.ingimage.com

This book is a translation from the original published under ISBN 978-620-5-50671-4.

Publisher:
Sciencia Scripts
is a trademark of
Dodo Books Indian Ocean Ltd. and OmniScriptum S.R.L publishing group

120 High Road, East Finchley, London, N2 9ED, United Kingdom
Str. Armeneasca 28/1, office 1, Chisinau MD-2012, Republic of Moldova, Europe
Printed at: see last page
ISBN: 978-620-6-07491-5

PREFACE

Pharmacy is an area of healthcare that has undergone major changes in recent decades, especially with regard to its clinical and multidisciplinary approach. Increasingly, pharmacists have taken on a prominent role in the healthcare team, working together with other professionals to ensure the safety and eficacy of drug therapy.The multidisciplinary approach in pharmacy aims to integrate different areas of knowledge and action, such as medicine, nursing, nutrition, fisioterapia, psychology, among others, in order to offer more complete and personalized care to patients. With this approach, it is possible to promote a broader and more integrated view of health, considering not only the use of medication, but also other relevant aspects, such as nutrition, lifestyle, mental and emotional health, among others.This book aims to present the multidisciplinary approach in pharmacy and its importance to clinical practice. Topics such as patient assessment, selection and prescription of medications, identification and prevention of adverse reactions, promotion of the rational use of medications, and monitoring of therapy over time will be addressed, always with an integrated and multidisciplinary approach.We believe that a multidisciplinary approach in pharmacy is essential for quality, safe and eficacious clinical practice. We hope this book will be a valuable source of information and guidance for all healthcare profissionals involved in drug therapy, contributing to more effective and patient-centered pharmaceutical care.

I dedicate this book to the pharmacists, pharmacy students, researchers, and profissionals from afins who work tirelessly to ensure the quality and safety of medicines and contribute to the advancement of pharmaceutical science. Their commitment and dedication to public health are inspiring and critical to ensuring a better future for us all.

AUTHORS

PROFª DRª GABRIELA CAVALCANTE DA SILVA

Master in Pharmaceutical Sciences (UFPE 2015.1) in the research line Obtaining and Evaluating Natural and Bioactive Products and PhD in Biochemistry and Physiology (UFPE 2020.1) developing research in toxicological evaluation and pharmacological application of protein concentrates and lectins. Professor at the Faculdade de Integração do Sertão (FIS) and Professor at the University of Pernambuco Medical School (Serra Talhada). Professor at the Post-Graduation of IDE and CEFAPP Group. Develops research in toxicological evaluation and pharmacological application of products, as well as in the area of drug consumption by the population. Experience and aptitude in the areas of Pharmacology, Toxicology, Physiology, Biochemistry and Pharmaceutical Assistance.

PROFº M.Sc. JOSÉ ISRAEL GUERRA JUNIOR

PhD candidate in the Postgraduate Program in Therapeutic Innovation (PPGIT) at the Federal University of Pernambuco (UFPE), in the research line of Design, Molecular Modeling and Preparation of Bioactive Products (2022-2026). He is Master in the Post-Graduation Program in Pharmaceutical Sciences (PPGCF) at the Federal University of Pernambuco (UFPE), in the research line of Obtaining and Evaluating Natural and Bioactive Products (2022-2026) Specialist in Clinical and Hospital Pharmacy at Unyleya College (2021). Graduated in Pharmacy (2019) from the University Center of the Ipojuca Valley (Unifavip | Wyden). He completed his secondary education (high school) at Queen Elizabeth Regional High School, Canada, through the Newfoundland International Education Program. He has experience in Microbiology, Pharmacognosy, Natural Products, Pharmacology and Toxicology. He is a professor in the Pharmacy, Nursing, Psychology, and Dentistry courses at the Maurício de Nassau University Center in Caruaru, and is a member of the Núcleo Docente Estruturante (NDE) of the Pharmacy course and member of the Pharmacy and Psychology courses' council. He also works as a post-graduation professor at IDE College and the Metropolitan College of Anapolis (FAMA). In the assistance part, he works as Clinical and Hospital Pharmacist at Unimed Caruaru and Assistant Pharmacist at Farmacia Trabalhador do Brasil.

SUMMARY

ANALYSIS OF POSSIBLE DRUG INTERACTIONS IN PRESCRIPTIONS OF ELDERLY HYPERTENSIVE PATIENTS IN A PRIMARY CARE UNIT HEALTH

¹ Pharmacy student, Faculdade de Integração do Sertão - FIS.
² PhD student at the Federal University of Pernambuco.
³ Professor at the University of Pernambuco and at the Faculdade de Integração do Sertão.
Ana Clara Leite Fernandes ¹ Rennan Luiz Leite Diniz ¹ José Israel Guerra Junior ² Gabriela Cavalcante da Silva ³

SUMMARY

Introduction: Hypertension is considered a chronic non-communicable disease, and is the main risk factor for cardiovascular morbidity and mortality in the geriatric population. Moreover, this public is prone to present other comorbidities, and therefore, to the concomitant use of several drugs, such act is identified as polypharmacy; the association of drugs when well used, optimizes the treatment and maximizes results, however, if done improperly can cause adverse reactions and drug interactions, bringing more complications to the health of those affected. Objective: To investigate the presence of polypharmacy and analyze the possible drug interactions present in the pharmacological prescriptions contained in the medical records of elderly hypertensive patients at the Umãs Basic Health Unit. Metodologia: Tratou-se de um estudo descritivo, transversal, com abordagem quanti-qualitativa, e teve com N amostral, 141 prontuários de hipertensos com idade igual ou superior a 60 anos. Results: It was possible to verify the presence of polypharmacy in 32.6% of the medical records, 54.3% of which were female; the drug interactions were classified according to their degree of risk: mild (8.6%), moderate (84.8%) and severe (6.5%). The most recurrent interactions happened between hydrochlorothiazide and the oral hypoglycemic agents, metformin and glibenclamide, both with moderate severity. Conclusion: The results found revealed a high prevalence of possible drug interactions in the studied population, reinforcing the need for a multiprofessional team, including the pharmacist, in primary care, in order to promote a safe, effective treatment that does not affect the patient's quality of life.

Keywords: Hypertension. Drug Interactions. Polypharmacy.

INTRODUCTION

Systemic Arterial Hypertension (SAH) is characterized by the persistent elevation of systolic and diastolic blood pressure (BP), and is considered a chronic noncommunicable disease (CNCD), resulting from the combination of several factors, such as genetic, environmental and sociocultural (BARROSO et al., 2020). According to estimates by the World Health Organization (WHO) (2013), chronic noncommunicable diseases (NCDs) are a health problem of great proportion and a serious public health problem. Among the most frequent chronic diseases, circulatory system diseases are the vast majority, being responsible for 17 million deaths/year worldwide. Deaths related to complications caused by systemic arterial hypertension (SAH) are the most prevalent, and account for 55.3% (WHO, 2013). Since the BP values considered normal for adults are 120 mmHg and 80 mmHg, systolic and diastolic, respectively, people who present systolic BP greater than or equal to 140 mmHg and/or diastolic BP greater than or equal to 90 mmHg, measured with the correct technique, on at least two occasions, without the use of antihypertensive drugs are considered hypertensive (BARROSO et al., 2020).According to the Brazilian Guidelines on Hypertension (2020) in the geriatric population, SAH is the main risk factor for cardiovascular morbidity and mortality, existing of hypertension in the population aged over 65 years, reaching more than 60%. According to Esperandio et al. (2013) and Gonçalves and Pereira (2021) there is much evidence that the elderly population has a greater vulnerability, made possible by physiological changes caused by the aging process itself, which makes them more prone to the development of chronic diseases, among them SAH, which is the main NCD in this population.It is worth noting that the elderly may have an average of three to five chronic diseases, requiring the use of more than one type of medication. This fact predisposes the occurrence of polypharmacy, which according to the Institute for Safe Medication Use Practices (ISMP) (2017) is defined as the concomitant use of four or more types of drugs, so the choice of antihypertensive should be guided based on the comorbidities that already exist in the patient, and should give priority to drugs that can also bring benefits to other diseases in order to avoid drug interactions (OLIVEIRA et al, 2021).

Drug interactions, as described by Jacomini and Silva (2011) are a clinical event where the effects of a drug are altered by the presence of another drug, food, drink or some chemical environmental agent. However, faced with the various difficulties of proving the real occurrence, studies are usually focused on the investigation of potential drug interactions (PDIs), that is, those interactions with possibilities of causing harm to the patient, already known and already documented in the (SANTOS; GIORDANI; ROSA, 2019).The therapeutic monitoring of an elderly hypertensive patient is of great value, since NCDs, including SAH, have high prevalence and are considered a challenge for Primary Health Care teams (SILVA, 2021). For the patient to follow the treatment correctly, according to Santos (2012), it is of utmost importance that health professionals know how to clarify the possible doubts presented, so that the patient follows the proposed recommendations and has adherence to treatment, being the pharmaceutical professional the most qualified for this task at the time of drug dispensation. Given the above, this study aimed to analyze the occurrence of polypharmacy and verify the frequency and degree of risk of possible drug interactions through the analysis of prescriptions contained in the medical records of elderly hypertensive patients, followed up in primary care, in order to promote the correct guidelines for the patient to use the medication in the best possible way through appropriate information, in order to advise and monitor the rational use of the drug ensuring its safety, avoiding complications arising from possible drug interactions and emphasizing the importance of the professional pharmacist in the multidisciplinary team.

METHODOLOGY

This was a descriptive, observational, cross-sectional, retrospective study with a quantitative and qualitative approach, developed with the objective of analyzing the prescriptions contained in the medical records of elderly hypertensive patients registered at the Umãs Basic Health Unit, in order to assess the presence and frequency of drug interactions and polypharmacy. The research was conducted in the UBS of Umãs, a district of Salgueiro, located in the hinterland of Pernambuco, 27.5 km from the city, where an average of 220 elderly patients are seen monthly. The research included all medical records of elderly patients with hypertension registered in the UBS, and who have access to medications in the mentioned unit.After approval by the Research Ethics Committee of the Faculdade de Integração do Sertão -FIS, CAAE number: 57603622.1.0000.8267 and opinion number: 033159/2022, a data survey was carried out between the months of May and June 2022, of all medical records of hypertensive individuals aged 60 years or older. The drug interactions were analyzed with the help of the Drugs Interactions Checker database, and were classified according to their degree of risk: mild, moderate, and severe. All medical records containing four or more medications were considered to have polypharmacy (ISMP, 2017).

The following variables were used as variables: age and gender of the patient, presence of polypharmacy, medications used, presence of other pathologies, and the identification of drug interactions. All data obtained in this study were thoroughly analyzed and processed as graphs using GraphPad Prism software, version 8.0.

RESULTS AND DISCUSSION

Aging consists of a biological process intrinsic to the nature of the human being, the presence of morphological, functional, biochemical, and psychological changes, bring to the individual's body a greater vulnerability and consequently a lower capacity to adapt and respond to the stresses of the environment, leading the elderly to have a greater propensity to develop chronic diseases (MARIA, 2017).In this study, 141 medical records of elderly hypertensive patients were analyzed, reaching the sample size of the research, considering 95% reliability and 5% error, a number obtained through the monthly flow of patients in the unit and considering the period of data collection. Among the participants, 51.1% (72) are between 60-70 years old, 32.6% (46) between 71-80 years old, 12.8% (18) between 81-90 years old, and 3.5% (5) are between 91-100 years old, graph 1. These findings corroborate the North American study where a prevalence of SAH of 62.25% was observed among 60-69 year olds. Unlike the results found in the study conducted by Menezes et. al, (2016), which had as sample elderly residents in the city of Campina Grande-PB, observing a prevalence of SAH of 81% among individuals aged 70-79 years.

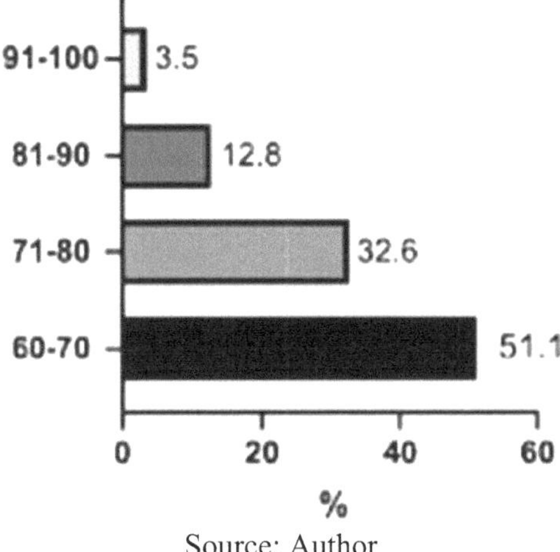

Graph 1 - Distribution of patients according to age range.

Source: Author

Non-adherence to drug treatment for SAH is a major problem and the main factor related to the inadequate control of blood pressure in the elderly population, which negatively affects the success of therapy and leads to further complications to the health of the affected person (SOUSA et. al., 2018). In a study conducted by Dantas and collaborators (2020), between the years 2012 and 2014, in a basic health unit in the state of Pará, about the prevalence of adherence to SAH treatment, 39 (62.9%) of 62 participants in the research did not maintain treatment.According to graph 2, 32.6% (46) of the medical records analyzed presented polypharmacy, which, according to the ISMP, is defined as the concomitant and continuous use of four or more medications (ISMP, 2017). The data presented are in agreement with a research conducted by Silva et al. (2021), in a basic health unit, in the state of Pará, with diabetic and/or hypertensive patients, where it was observed a predominance of elderly people over 60 years old (67.3%) in use of polypharmacy. Polypharmacy was also expressed in a study conducted in Porto Velho-RO in a family health unit with 87 elderly, where 34.5% of the participants' prescriptions were in this condition (FARIAS and RODRIGUES, 2022).

Graph 2 - Percentage of medical records with the presence of polypharmacy.

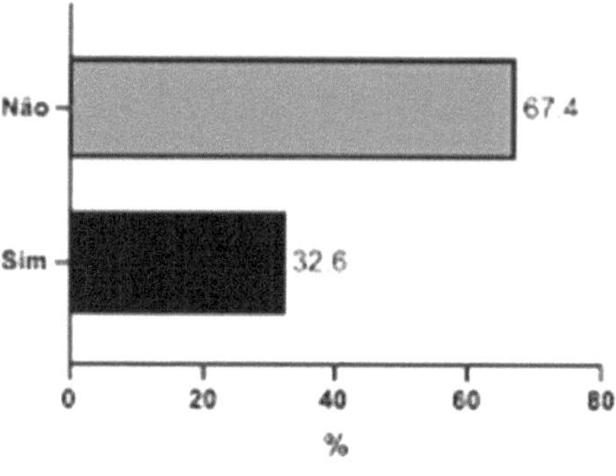

Source: Author

Polypharmacy is present at all ages, however, it is still predominant in the elderly population, as well as in patients with comorbidities and among the main risks presented to this public are sedation, delirium, gastrointestinal bleeding, falls, fractures, drug interactions, low adherence to the prescribed treatment, hospitalizations, Potentially Inappropriate Prescription (PIP) and death (GONÇALVES, OLIVEIRA, REIS, 2022). According to the surveyed data, among the medical records identified with polypharmacy, 54.3% (25) belonged to the female gender and 45.6% (21) to the male gender (Graph 3). Such results are due to the fact that women are more concerned about their health, and for biological reasons are more likely to present comorbidities, as well as use health services more often when compared to men (LIMA et al., 2016).

Graph 3 - Distribution of patients with polypharmacy according to gender.

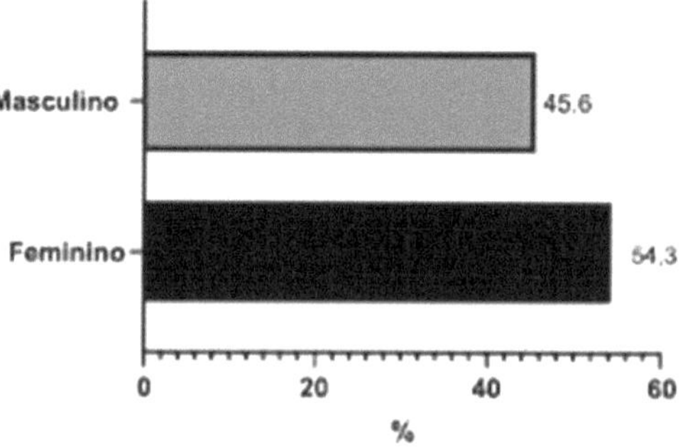

Source: Author

Brazil has been going through an accelerated and growing population aging process, such fact explains the rising prevalence of adults and elderly with NCDs, and consequently, there is an increase in the use of multiple medications (PIO et al. 2021). Among the 46 medical records found of patients who are in polypharmacy, 95.65% (44) present other comorbidities, among which we can highlight hyperlipidemia, diabetes mellitus, cardiovascular diseases, joint pathologies and depression. In a study conducted with hypertensive patients in São Luís- MA, by Monteiro et al., (2015), it was possible to observe that in addition to SAH, 3.33% of respondents reported heart disease, 3.33% panic syndrome, 5% rheumatic disease, 8.33% osteopenia, 1.67% cancer and 56.67% diabetes mellitus.The drug therapy for hypertension is usually initiated with the use of a single drug, however, most hypertensive patients do not achieve optimal BP control with a single therapeutic agent, requiring the association with other pharmacological classes (GEWEHR, et al. 2018). According to Monteiro et al. (2015) the concomitant use of two antihypertensives, when well used, can cause drug synergism, increasing the chance of success in BP control. In most of the medical records analyzed, it was possible to identify some type of drug interaction, using as computerized database, Drugs Interaction Checker, the interactions were classified according to the degree of risk (minimal, moderate, and high risk). In total, 86.5% (122) medical records were identified with the presence of MI, of these, 8.6% (21) were considered as mild, 84.8% (244) were moderate, and 6.5% (16) were considered as severe, as can be seen in graph 4. In the study conducted by Silva (2020), in the city of Afogados da Ingazeira, it was possible to observe the presence of drug interactions in 31.3% (87) of prescriptions for the elderly, 28.7% (25) being severe, 71.3% (62) moderate, and only 1.1% (1) considered as mild, partially agreeing with the present study. In turn, Gotardelo et al. (2014) in Minas Gerais, with 273 elderly, demonstrated a prevalence of 55.6% of potential drug interactions, of which 5.6% were mild, 81.6% were moderate and 12.8% were of greater severity, with this higher frequency of moderate interactions as well as the cited studies.

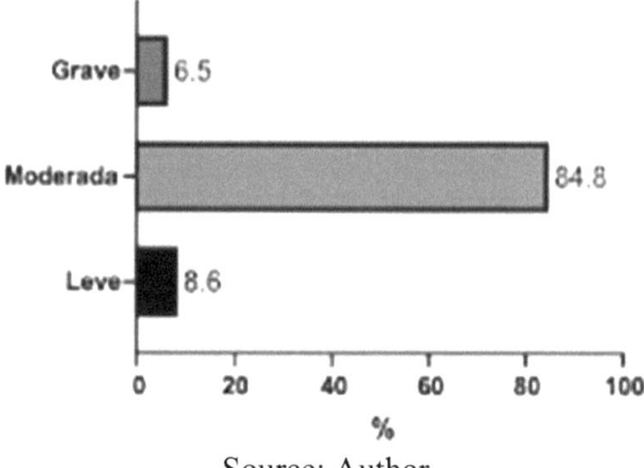

Source: Author

In table 1 we can see the most frequent MI found in the analyzed medical records, which occurred among different classes of antihypertensives, non-steroidal anti-inflammatory drugs (NSAIDs), and oral hypoglycemic agents.

Table 1 - Most frequent drug interactions.

Serious Interactions		Frequency
Losartana	Spironolactone	3 (18,7%)
Losartana	Captopril	2 (12,5%)
Losartana	Enalapril	2 (12,5%)
Moderate Interactions		
Hydrochlorothiazide	Metformin	22 (10,6%)
Hydrochlorothiazide	Glibenclamide	14 (6,8%)
Losartana	AAS	13 (6,3%)
Mild Interactions		
Hydrochlorothiazide	Anlodipine	3 (14,3%)
Atenolol	AAS	2 (9,5%)

Source: Author

Drug interactions can be described as a clinical event, which occurs from the co-administration of a drug with other drugs, food or other chemical substances, and that can alter its effectiveness leading to an increase or decrease in its pharmacological action (SILVA, 2020). According to Santos, Giordani, and Rosa (2019), the studies on MI are focused on the investigation of Potential Drug Interactions (PDIs), i.e., those that are already identified in the literature as harmful to the patient's health.The study conducted by Silva (2021), in the city of Serra Talhada, where the presence of drug interactions in the prescriptions of hypertensive patients was analyzed, also showed that the highest frequency of interactions was found among different classes of antihypertensives, non-steroidal anti-inflammatory drugs (NSAIDs), and oral hypoglycemic agents.

Among the mild MI identified in the current study, the two most prevalent were between, Hydrochlorothiazide and Anlodipine, and between Atenolol and ASA corresponding to 14.2% (3) and 9.5% (2) of the mild interactions, respectively. Hydrochlorothiazide is part of the class of thiazide diuretics, and is widely used in the treatment of AH, alone or in combination. Its mechanism of action causes an increase in urinary output (mainly of sodium and water), and consequently, with increased diuresis, the volume of extracellular fluid is decreased along with blood pressure (COSTA and ABREU, 2021). Anlodipine belongs to the class of calcium channel blockers, and when associated with Hydrochlorothiazide may cause renal dysfunction, depending on how long the patient uses this combination (SILVA, 2021). Although some drug associations are planned, the geriatric patient needs more attention when compared to others, since the physiological decline caused by advanced age can induce the development of different adverse reactions (OLIVEIRA et al., 2020).Acetylsalicylic acid (ASA) belongs to the class of nonsteroidal anti-inflammatory drugs (NSAIDs), and is widely used by the geriatric population as a platelet antiaggregant in order to prevent cardiovascular diseases. When associated with Betablockers, such as Atenolol, it can reduce the antihypertensive capacity of the drug, due to the inhibition of renal prostaglandins, causing damage to blood pressure control (MAIA; FREITAS, 2021).According to table 1, the moderate drug interactions correspond to 84.8% (244) of all drug interactions found in the analyzed medical records. associations that appeared in greater proportion: Hydrochlorothiazide and Metformin with prevalence of 10.6% (22), followed by Hydrochlorothiazide and Glibenclamide with 6.7% (14), and lastly ASA and Losartan representing 6.2% (13). Such findings corroborate the results of a study by Leão et al. (2020), with hypertensive patients in the city of Jequié-BA, where the highest occurrence of MI were between Hydrochlorothiazide and Glibenclamide (11.45%) and Hydrochlorothiazide and Metformin (10.89%), both considered moderate severity.Among the most frequent moderate MI, the use of Hydrochlorothiazide with oral hypoglycemic agents, such as Metformin, a biguanide that acts by reducing insulin resistance, decreasing the hepatic production of glucose and increasing the uptake of glucose and its utilization by the tissues, and with Glibenclamide, a sulfonylurea whose mechanism is the stimulation of insulin secretion by the beta cells of the pancreas (SAKAJI,

VINICIUS TOSHIO, 2022), stands out. The associations of hydrochlorothiazide with the hypoglycemic agents mentioned, according to Andrade and Souza (2018) have a pharmacokinetic character and occur due to a mechanism induced by diuretics, which causes an alteration in glucose tolerance, as well as in its metabolization, such mechanisms can lead to a lack of glycemic control, increasing the risks of hyperglycemia (LEÃO et al., 2020).The simultaneous administration of ASA and Losartan is also classified as moderate risk, appearing in 6.2% (13) of medical records. According to the Brazilian Guidelines on Hypertension (2010), the antihypertensive mechanism of Losartan consists in antagonizing the action of angiotensin II, promoting smooth muscle relaxation, besides increasing the renal excretion of water and sodium. The coadministration of ASA with Losartan, may cause an increase in blood pressure as a result of inhibition of renal synthesis of prostaglandins or by retention of organic fluids and sodium, caused by ASAs, such mechanisms may antagonize the effects of Losartan, as well as of most antihypertensives, so dose adjustments and more effective monitoring of these patients may be valid strategies (JACKELINE, 2018).The most recurrent interaction classified as of greater severity happened between Losartan and Spironolactone, corresponding to 18.7% (3). Spironolactone competitively inhibits aldosterone receptors, resulting in diuretic and antihypertensive effects due to a greater excretion of sodium and water (AMARO, 2020). The concomitant use of these drugs may increase the risk of hyperkalemia. Elderly patients and/or patients with other diseases, such as diabetes mellitus, kidney and heart problems, are part of the risk group and are even more prone to develop hyperkalemia.Hyperkalemia, which can progress from mild symptoms such as nausea, vomiting, and weakness to kidney failure, muscle paralysis, changes in heart rhythm, and cardiac arrest (DRUGS INTERACTIONS, 2022).Another MI detected is considered serious, was between Losartan and the Angiotensin Converting Enzyme Inhibitors (ACEI's), Captopril and Enalapril, both representing 12.5% (2). The association between these two pharmacological classes has synergistic effects on the renin-angiotensin system, and is linked to the risk of hyperkalemia and renal dysfunction, requiring the monitoring of BP, renal function and electrolytes (MONTEIRO et al., 2015).Similar data were observed in the study conducted by Cavalcante (2019), with elderly hypertensive patients in the city of Fortaleza-CE, where drug interactions classified as severe had a percentage of 4.86%, the moderate had a percentage of 81.59%, and as well as in the current study having the highest prevalence among diuretics. with hypoglycemic agents (18.75%).Results obtained by Alves and collaborators (2019) about drug interactions between antihypertensives and oral hypoglycemic agents in the city of Juazeiro do Norte-CE corroborate the present study, where most of the interactions found were of moderate clinical relevance with a higher frequency of interaction between Metformin and Hydrochlorothiazide, representing 61.54%.

CONCLUSION

The results obtained showed a high prevalence of drug interactions and polypharmacy in the population studied, and from this perspective, the need for special attention focused on the elderly hypertensive patient is highlighted, as well as the pharmacotherapeutic follow-up of this public, since the presence of drug interactions is an eminent risk, especially in the elderly and polymedicated patients. The use of tools to check drug interactions by health professionals is of great value, in order to promote a more comprehensive view of the patient's pharmacotherapy, besides emphasizing the importance of multidisciplinary work in primary care, in order to maximize positive therapeutic outcomes and thus contribute to the safety and quality of life of the individual.

REFERENCES

ALVES, N. R.; et al. Evaluation of drug interactions between antihypertensive and oral hypoglycemic agents/Evaluation of drug interactions between antihypertensive and oral hypoglycemic agents. **Journal of Psychology**, v. 13, n. 44, p. 374-392, 2019. Available at: https://doi.org/10.14295/idonline.v13i44.1625 Accessed: 15 May 2022.

AMARO, J. M. C. **Effects of spironolactone at the vascular level**. 2020. Doctoral Thesis. Available at: http://hdl.handle.net/10400.6/10646 Accessed on: May 15, 2022.

ANDRADE, K. V. F. de; SOUZA, A. M. Prevalence of potential drug interactions in hypertensive individuals followed-up in the health care strategy of the family. **Journal of Health & Biological Sciences**, v. 6, n. 4, p. 405-411, 2018. Available at: http://dx.doi.org/10.12662/2317-3076jhbs.v6i4.2090.p405-411.2018 Accessed on: 25 May 2022.

ANDRADE, N. de O.; ALVES, A. M.; LUCHESI, B. M.; MARTINS, T. C. R. Polymedication in adults and elderly enrolled in the Family Health Strategy: association with sociodemographic factors, lifestyle, social support network and health. **Revista Brasileira de Medicina de Família e Comunidade**, Rio de

Janeiro, v. 15, n. 42, p. 2462, 2020. Available at:
https://rbmfc.emnuvens.com.br/rbmfc/article/view/2462. Accessed on: 18 May
2022.

BARROSO, W. K.S., et al. Diretrizes brasileiras de hipertensão arterial-2020.
Arq Bras Cardiol. 2021; 116(3):516-658.Available at:
<https://www.scielo.br/j/abc/a/Z6m5gGNQCvrW3WLV7csqbqh/?format=pdf&la
ng=pt>A ces so on: September 28, 2021.

CAVALCANTE, V. C. **Analysis of drug interactions in elderly hypertensive
patients seen at a community pharmacy in the city of Fortaleza, Ceará**. 29f.
Article (Undergraduate in Pharmacy) - Fametro University Center, Fortaleza,
2019. [Advisor: Ma. Patrícia Fernandes da Silveira]. Available at:
http://repositorio.fametro.com.br/jspui/handle/123456789/939 Accessed on: 15
May 2022.

COSTA, J. J. de L.; ABREU, T. P. Effects of losartan with hydrochlorothiazide
combination therapy in patients of the popular pharmacy program. **Revista
Ibero-Americana de Humanidades, Ciências e Educação,** v. 7, n. 10, p. 1266-
1275, 2021. Available at: https://doi.org/10.51891/rease.v7i10.2660 Accessed
on: 14 May 2022.

CUTLER, J. A. et al. Trends in prevalence, awareness, treatment, and control
rates of hypertension in United States adults between 1988-1994 and 1999-
2004. **Hipertensão**. 2008;52(5):818 827. Available
at:10.1161/HIPERTENSONAHA.108.113357 Accessed May 12, 2022.

DANTAS, K. R. G. et al. Hypertensão arterial sistêmica: prevalência da adesão
ao tratamento em uma unidade de saúde do Pará. **Revista Eletrônica Acervo
Científico**. v. 11, p. e3978, 6 Aug. 2020. Available at:
https://doi.org/10.25248/reac.e3978.2020 Accessed on: 15 May 2022.

DRUGS. Drugs interactions Checker. **Drugs.com**. Last updated: 16-05-2022.
Available at: https://www.drugs.com/drug_interactions.html. Accessed May 20,
2022.

ESPERANDIO, E. M.; et al . Prevalence and factors associated with
hypertension in the elderly in municipalities of Amazônia Legal, MT. **Rev.
bras. geriatr. gerontol.**, Rio de Janeiro , v. 16, n. 3, p. 481-493, Sept. 2013.
Available at: SciELO - Brazil - Prevalence and factors associated with
hypertension in the elderly in municipalities of the Legal Amazon, MT
Prevalence and factors associated with hypertension in the elderly in
municipalities of the Legal Amazon, MT Accessed on: 29 September 2021.

FARIAS, N de A. S. RODRIGUES, R. V. The influence of polypharmacy in elderly people enrolled in a family health unit in Porto Velho - RO. Brazilian Journal of Development. Curitiba, v.8, n.4, p. 27459-27488, apr., 2022. Available at: https://doi.org/10.34117/bjdv8n4-310 Accessed on: May 13, 2022.

SAKAJI, VINICIUS TOSHIO. The Role of the Pharmacist in the Care of the Diabetic Patient. Unesp.br, 2022. Accessed on: 20 February 2023.

GEWEHR, D. M. et al. Adherence to pharmacological treatment of hypertension in Primary Health Care. Saúde em Debate. Rio de Janeiro, v. 42, n 116, p. 179-190, 2018. Available at: https://doi.org/10.1590/0103-1104201811614 Accessed on: 13 May 2022.

GONÇALVES, D; PEREIRA, R. M. Análise de possíveis interações medicamentosas em prescrições para idosos hipertensos. Brazilian Journal of Development, v.7, n. 4, 2021. Available at: 27845-71487-1-PB.pdf Accessed on: September 29, 2021.

GONÇALVES, M. H. A. DE F.; OLIVEIRAC, R. V.; REIS, B. C. C. Polypharmacy and the

elderly population in Primary Health Care: a literature review. Revista Eletrônica Acervo Médico, v. 3, p. e9777, 21 fev. 2022. Available at: https://doi.org/10.25248/reamed.e9777.2022 Accessed on: 13 May 2022.

GOTARDELO, D. R. et al. Prevalence and factors associated with potential drug interactions among the elderly in a population-based study. Rev Bras Med Fam Comunidade. Rio de Janiero; v 9(31):111-8.2014. Available at: http://dx.doi.org/10.5712/rbmfc9(31)833 Accessed on: 14 May 2022.

JACOMINI, L. C. L. SILVA, N. A. D. Interações medicamentosas: uma contribuição para o uso racional de imunossupressores sintéticos e biológicos. Revista Brasileira de Reumatologia, v. 51, n. 2, p. 168-174, 2011. Available at: SciELO - Brazil - Drug interactions: a contribution to the rational use of synthetic and biological immunosuppressants Drug interactions: a contribution to the rational use of synthetic and biological immunosuppressants. Access on: October 1st, 2021.

LEÃO, I. N. et al. Prevalência das interações medicamentosas potenciais em hipertensos atendidos na atenção primária. Revista de Atenção à Saúde. São Caetano do Sul, v. 18, n. 63, p. 05-13, jan./mar., 2020. Available at: https://doi.org/10.13037/ras.vol18n63.6031 Accessed on: 14 May 2022.

LIMA, T. A. M. et al. Analysis of potential drug interactions and adverse reactions to nonsteroidal anti-inflammatory drugs in the elderly. **Revista Bras. Geriatr. Gerontol**. Rio de Janeiro, v 19(3):533-544. 2016. Available at: https://doi.org/10.1590/1809-98232016019.150062 Accessed on: 18 May 2022.

MAIA, A. P. A. FREITAS, L. T. Hipertensão arterial e possíveis interações medicamentosas: Um olhar atento do farmacêutico no cuidado ao idoso. **Brazilian Journal of Development**.

Curitiba, v. 7, n. 5, p. 48245-48255, 2021. Available at: https://doi.org/10.34117/bjdv.v7i5.29746 Accessed on: May 14, 2022.

MENEZES, T. N. Prevalence and control of hypertension in the elderly: a population-based study. **Portuguese Journal of Public Health**. 2016; v 34(2):117-124. Available at: https://doi.org/10.1016/j.rpsp.2016.04.001 Accessed on: 11 May 2022.

SANTOS, J. DA S.; GIORDANI, F.; ROSA, M. L. G. Potential drug interactions in adults and the elderly in primary care. **Ciência & Saúde Coletiva**, v. 24, n. 11, p. 4335-4344, nov. 2019. Accessed on: 20 February 2023.

MONTEIRO, S. C. M. et al. Study of potential drug interactions in hypertensive patients. **Infarma-Pharmaceutical Sciences**, v. 27, n. 2, p. 117-125, 2015. Available at: 723-3658-1-PB.pdf Accessed on: 15 May 2022.

NASCIMENTO, R. C. R. M.; et al. Polifarmácia: uma realidade na atenção primária do Sistema Único de Saúde. **Rev. Saúde Pública** [online]. Brazil, v.51, suppl.2, 19s.
November. 2017. Available at:
https://www.scielo.br/j/rsp/a/xMVtMdQ7pdM7zcGSVFBMrdm/?format=pdf&lang=pt Accessed on: September 30, 2021

OLIVEIRA, F. M. R. L. et al. Syndrome of the frail elderly: conceptual analysis according to Walker and Avant. **Revista Brasileira de Enfermagem**, v. 73 (Suppl 3), 2020. Available at: https://doi.org/10.1590/0034-7167-2019-0601 Accessed on: 06 June 2022.

OLIVEIRA, P. C. et al. Prevalence and Factors Associated with Polypharmacy in Elderly Patients Attended in Primary Health Care in Belo Horizonte-MG, **Brazil. Ciência & Saúde Coletiva**, 26(4):1553-1564, April 2021. Available at: https://www.scielo.br/j/csc/a/hqJVhghhLCxp6mFSFsWFdYH/?format=pdf&lang=pt Accessed on: September 29, 2021

PIO, G. P. ALEXANDRE, P. R F. TOLEDO, L. F. S. Polypharmacy and risks in the elderly population. **Brazilian Journal of Health Review**. Curitiba, v.4, n.2, p. 8924-8939 mar./apr. 2021. Available at: https://doi.org/10.34119/bjhrv4n2-403 Accessed on: May 13, 2022.

JACKELINE, S. Profile and management of drug interactions on hospital admission. **App.uff.br**, 2018. Accessed on: 20 February 2023.

SANTOS, J. da S.; GIORDANI, F.; ROSA, M. L. G. Potential drug interactions in adults and the elderly in primary care. **Ciência & Saúde Coletiva**, v. 24, p. 4335-4344, 2019. Available at: https://doi.org/10.1590/1413-812320182411.04692018 Accessed on: 14 May 2022.

SILVA, A. C. B. da. et al. Polypharmacy among hypertensive and diabetic patients in a health care unit. **Revista Eletrônica Acervo Saúde**, v. 13, n. 8, p. e8006, 7 Aug. 2021. Available at: https://doi.org/10.25248/reas.e8006.2021 Accessed on: 13 May 2022.

SILVA, L. G. FREQUENCY OF POLYPHARMACY AND POSSIBLE DRUG INTERACTIONS IN HYPERTENSIVE PATIENTS IN A BASIC HEALTH CARE UNIT OF THE CITY OF SÃO PAULO SERRA TALHADA. 2021. 16 f. Course Completion Paper (Bachelor's Degree in Pharmacy) - Faculdade de Integração do Sertão, Serra Talhada, 2021. [Advisor: Profª. Drª. Gabriela Cavalcante da Silva.]

MARIA. Aging, social network and functionality in daily life : A study in Day Centers and Senior University of Guimarães. **241.119**, 2017. Accessed on: 20 February 2023.

SILVA, Y. B. PHARMACOTHERAPY PROFILE IN PRESCRIPTIONS OF A POPULATION

ELDERLY WOMAN SERVED IN A BASIC PHARMACY.2020. 18 f. Course Completion Paper (Bachelor's Degree in Pharmacy) - Faculdade de Integração do Sertão, Serra Talhada, 2020. [Advisor: Profª. Drª. Gabriela Cavalcante da Silva].

SOCIEDADE BRASILEIRA DE CARDIOLOGIA.VI Diretrizes Brasileiras de Hipertensão. **Arq Bras Cardiol** 2010; 95: 1-51. Available at: Diretriz_hipertensao_associados.pdf (cardiol.br) Accessed on: 29 September 2021.

SOUSA, R. C. et al. Particularities of elderly hypertensive patients to drug treatment adherence. **Rev Enferm UFPE** [online]. Recife, 12(1):216-23, jan., 2018. Available at: https://doi.org/10.5205/1981-8963-v12i01a23296p216-223-2018 Accessed on: May 12, 2022.

WORLD HEALTH ORGANIZATION. **A global brief on hypertension**: silent killer, global public health crisis. World Health Day 2013. Geneva: World Health Organization; 2013.Available at:< W (who.int)> Accessed on: 28 September 2021

WORLD HEALTH ORGANIZATION**. Medication Without Harm - Global Patient Safety Challenge on Medication Safety.** Geneva: World Health Organization, 2017. Available at: ISMP (ismp-brasil.org) Accessed on: 15 May 2022.

PROFILE OF PATIENT CONSUMPTION AND ERRORS IN ANTIDEPRESSANT PRESCRIPTIONS SEEN AT A PRIVATE PHARMACY IN HINTERLAND OF PERNAMBUCO

Leticia Valeska Rael Santana de Menezes [1]

José Israel Guerra Junior [2] *Gabriela Cavalcante da Silva* [3]

[1] *Pharmacy student, Faculdade de Integração do Sertão - FIS.*

[2] *PhD student at the Federal University of Pernambuco.*

[3] *Professor at the University of Pernambuco and at the Faculdade de Integração do Sertão.*

SUMMARY

Introduction: Antidepressants are psychiatric drugs that act on the central nervous system (CNS), widely used for the treatment of mental disorders such as depression, anxiety, addictions, sleep disorders, among others. Their period of use should not exceed as recommended, because they can cause several damages to the organism. **Objective: to** design an intervention project to control the use of antidepressants and possible prescription errors present in a private pharmacy in Custódia. **Methodology:** a questionnaire for data collection was carried out, via Google form, according to the needs in order to recognize the population described, considering age range, gender, comorbidities, among others, in addition to analyzing the fulfillment of the requirements of the prescriptions filled. **Results:** 178 prescriptions were analyzed, where it was observed the prevalence of the female gender (70.8%) with complete higher education (43.3%). As for the prescriptions and the correct filling of the prescription, the absence of date (25.8%), pharmaceutical form (39.3%), concentration (56.2%) and posology (30.3%) was verified. **Conclusion:** It was observed the need for awareness of prescribers in relation to rational prescription, as well as the need for orientation by the pharmacist to users.

Password: Antidepressants. Prescription Drugs. Medication Use

INTRODUCTION

Mental disorders comprise depression, anxiety disorder, bipolar disorder, schizophrenia, and others, characterized by many different symptoms. However, they are usually described by some abnormal thoughts, emotions, behaviors, and personal relationships. Examples of these disorders are schizophrenia, depression, intellectual disability, and disorders due to drug abuse (WHO, 2016). The aspects related to mental health have been the subject of great questions and changes in the ways of observing the whole population affected by psychic disturbances. The use of drugs with proven effectiveness in psychiatric disorders has become widespread since the mid-1950s. Today, between 10-15% of prescriptions in the United States are for drugs indicated to affect mental processes, such as: to sedate, stimulate, or in some way change mood, reasoning, or behavior (ROCHA, 2013).Antidepressants are the most frequently used treatment for remission or control of mental disorders. Some factors may adversely affect antidepressant therapy and significantly interfere with treatment adherence. Among these, we highlight the patient's level of education, the absence of information in the prescriptions, the information provided by the physician, the conflict between the therapeutic proposal and the patient's own behavior (MARQUES, 2012).Prescriptions play an important role in preventing medication errors (FERRARI et al., 2013). Incomplete, illegible, or erased prescriptions prevent the correct interpretation in the dispensation of medications, and can hinder the actions of pharmaceutical assistance and consequently compromise their pharmacotherapeutic treatment. The ideal is that prescriptions for the treatment of depression be produced by a specialist in psychiatry, neurology, or similar. The absence of these professionals can compromise the quality of the prescription of antidepressant medications, resulting from a wrong diagnosis, leading to unnecessary use of centrally acting medications (AZEVEDO, 2011).When dispensing drugs subject to special control, the presence of the pharmaceutical professional is indispensable, not only to prevent dispensing errors and reduce the costs of dispensing drugs. abuse, as well as to guide more effectively such patients who need more attention because they present a debilitated emotional state, that is, pharmaceutical assistance becomes fundamental to obtain the desired therapeutic results. The lack of information about medicines (pharmaceutical form, dosage, presentation) and their mode of use (posology, route of administration, treatment time) can lead to waste, pharmacotherapeutic loss and inadequate or undesired treatments (WAGNER; ANDRADE et al, 2010).It is important to note that the irrational and unmonitored use of antidepressant medications can lead to iatrogenesis, negative effects on the patient or complications resulting from any procedure performed by a health professional, and even mortality, in case of toxic doses (FERRARI, 2013; AZEVEDO et al., 2011). Medications are appointed as one of the main responsible for cases of poisoning, as well as occurrences in emergencies, hospitalizations in medical centers, and deaths. In 2017, SINITOX recorded about 20,637 cases of drug intoxication throughout Brazil, with the occurrence of 8,807 cases in children and adolescents aged 0 to 15 years. Children represent a group that is very susceptible to poisoning due to their psychological immaturity (FIOCRUZ, 2017).This study aimed to identify the profile of antidepressant users and analyze the possible errors in prescriptions dispensed in a private pharmacy in Custódia - PE, in order to demonstrate with this survey the risks and factors that predispose to abusive and prolonged use, thus providing necessary information to users and health professionals, especially to prescribers on prescription errors, dependence and long-term adverse effects, contributing to a better quality of life of patients.

MATERIALS AND METHODS

This was a field survey study carried out in the Municipality of Custódia, located in the hinterland of Pernambuco, specifically in the Pharmacy Rodrigues Pereira, where about 200 patients are assisted per month. The population was composed of 178 patients seen at the pharmacy with antidepressant prescriptions from public or private health services, who agreed to the research objectives, duly signing the Informed Consent Form (ICF). (ANNEX A). As selection criteria, prescriptions were excluded, as well as patients under 18 years of age and those who did not sign the ICF. Variables such as gender, education level, profession, legibility of the prescription, time of drug use, description of pharmaceutical form, prescriber's specialty, and date of prescription, among others, were determined.Data were collected through an online questionnaire on Google Form containing objective questions about the use of antidepressants, duration of treatment, mode of use, concomitant administration of other medications, among others, in clear language. The information collected from patients and antidepressant prescriptions were entered and analyzed in GraphPad Prism software version 8.0 spreadsheets, where graphs were constructed for better illustration and interpretation of the data.Since this is a research involving human beings, the researcher committed to obey the legal ethical aspects according to Resolutions Nº466/2012 and 510/2016 of the Regional Health Council that provides guidelines and regulatory standards for research on human beings. The project was forwarded and approved by the Research Ethics Committee of the Faculdade de Integração do Sertão - FIS, CAAE number: 34112720.0.0000.8267 and opinion: 4.314.214

RESULTS AND DISCUSSION

According to the WHO, at least two out of every twelve people on the planet suffer from mental health problems. Despite the consequences of this morbidity, only 1% of health professionals work in this area. In this context, pharmaceutical professionals are a considerable source for assessing patients with mental illness, ensuring the rational use and efficiency of pharmacological treatment. This professional can have a significant influence generating a link of care with mental health patients providing from basic guidelines to clinical services (CANADIAN PHARMACISTS ASSOCIATION, 2015).A total of 178 prescriptions were collected, within the study population 70.8% (126) were female and 29.2% (52) were male, showing a predominance of females in the treatment with antidepressants (Graph 1A). Rocha and Werlang (2013), also observed that women use antidepressants more than men, and that the increase in the consumption of antidepressants by women may be related to the prevalence of psychiatric disorders analyzed among people of this gender, besides the fact that they are more concerned about their health condition and attend health services more often. Women are two to three times more affected by depression than men and find it easier to accept that they are depressed and seek support (OLIVEIRA et al, 2012).

Chart 1- Distribution of patients using antidepressants according to gender (A) and education (B)

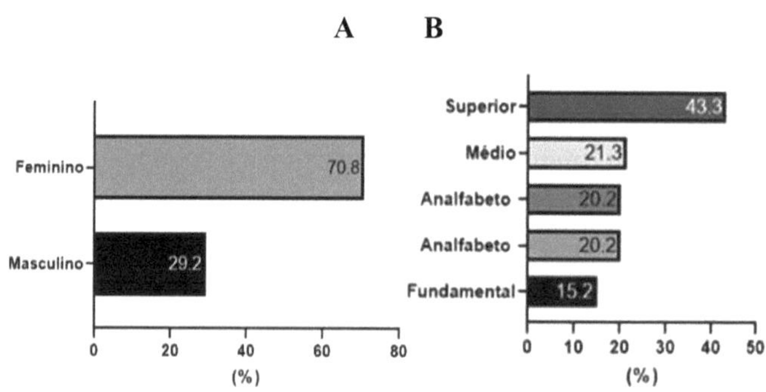

Source: Author

Other reasons that can justify the higher frequency of women as users of antidepressants are work problems, insomnia, and escape from problems (SOUZA, 2013). According to Pinho and Araújo (2012), this fact is correlated to the fact that women are given an overload of exhausting activities such as care and dedication to the home, raising children, household chores, and in some cases extra jobs to help with the monthly income.As illustrated in graph 1B, 21.3% (38) of the participants have high school education, 43.3% (77) higher education, 15.2%(27) elementary school, 20.2%(36) did not study. The higher rate of antidepressant use among patients with higher education with high school education, correlates to the fact that individuals with higher education invest more in their well-being and a greater demand for diagnosis, because they are the ones who most seek health services, for medical consultations for prevention and treatment (STOPA et al., 2015).On the other hand, Andrade et al., (2018), identified patients with elementary school education or who had no education, together totaling 35.4% of respondents as the most prevalent in the use of antidepressants. Due to little knowledge about antidepressants these may have greater difficulty understanding the risks, adverse and side effects of the medications which is a disadvantage for these users. General practitioner was the most frequent prescribing professional in this study, equivalent to more than half of the prescriptions analyzed 56.5%(100), followed by the specialties of psychiatrist 23.7% (42), rheumatologist 2.8%(5), cardiologist 5.1%(9), dermatologist 1.1%(2), neurologist 4.5%(8), orthopedist 1.7%(3), endocrinologist 1.1%(2), and 3.4% (6) did not have the prescriber's stamp (Graph 2). It would be expected that professionals such as neurologists or psychiatrists may be a more representative class in prescribing mental health medications, as these hold more specific knowledge of the pharmacological characteristics of this class of medications, as well as the pathological characteristics of patients (FERRARI, et al. 2013). Although clinical physicians understand less about the clinical, long-term effects and harms of these medications, they prescribe them comprehensively (ANTHIERENS et al., 2010).

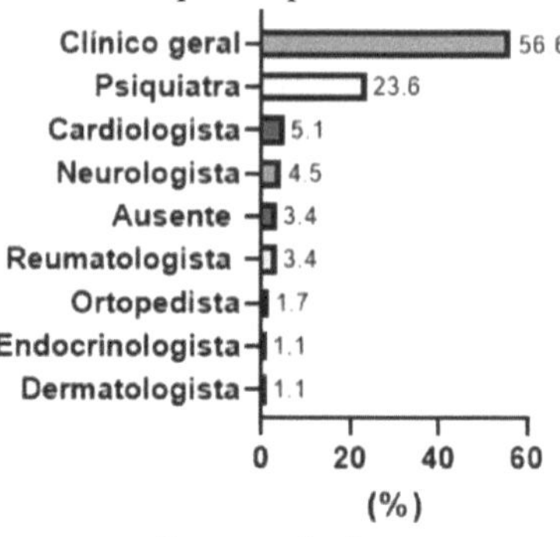

Chart 2 - Medical specialties of the professionals writing the antidepressant prescriptions

Source: Author

In 06 prescriptions analyzed it was not possible to observe the medical specialization, because only the prescriber's signature was present; such prescriptions could not be dispensed. Resolution No. 1931/09 of the Federal Council of Medicine prevents physicians from prescribing, attesting, or issuing reports, without proper identification of their registration number in the Regional Council of Medicine of their jurisdiction (CFM, 2009) Oliveira, Santos, and Leite (2015) cited that, in their research, 12.1% of the prescriptions did not contain the identification of the prescriber, i.e., the prescriber's stamp and/or signature were missing. Silva, Bandeira, and Oliveira (2012) stated that 15.3% of prescriptions were without the professional's stamp and 1% did not have the professional's signature. As illustrated in graph 3 below 67.4% (120) of the prescriptions were classified as readable, that is, there were no problems of time spent, beyond normal, to understand what was written, these results were higher than those found by Lucas et al (2012), when analyzing prescriptions of antidepressants filled in a private drugstore, identified a percentage of 22.5% (58) of illegible prescriptions.

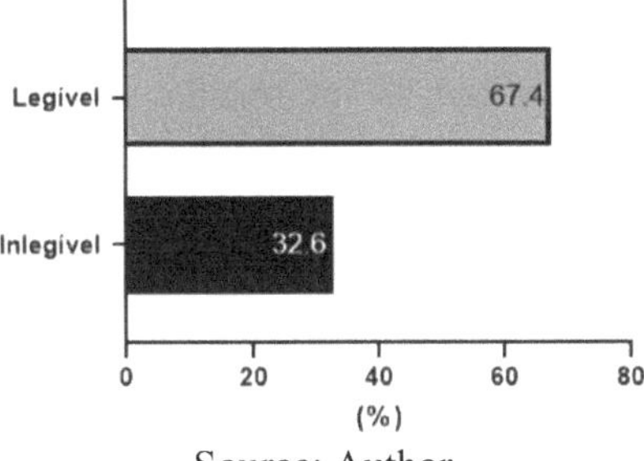

Graph 3 - Legibility of dispensed antidepressant prescriptions

Source: Author

The difficulty of legibility of the prescription and responsible for serious health problems, even classified as a lack of medical ethics. The dispensing of prescriptions under these conditions can lead to errors, with the probability of not achieving the desired therapeutic effect. In order for the patient's treatment to be effective, it is necessary that the medical prescription presents all the information identifying the drug, the patient and the prescriber, contributing to a safe dispensing, ensuring the quality and effectiveness of treatment (FIRMO et al., 2013).In view of the data collected, among the main errors detected is the lack of date on the prescription, 74.2% (132) had the date on the prescription and in 25.8% (46) did not included the date of the prescription (Graph 4 A). When the date of issue is not included in the prescription, it may contribute to the patient not having immediately used the prescribed medication, which may cause changes in symptoms (SOARES, 2014).

Graph 4 - Distribution of prescriptions according to the presence of issue date (A) and pharmaceutical form (B).

A B

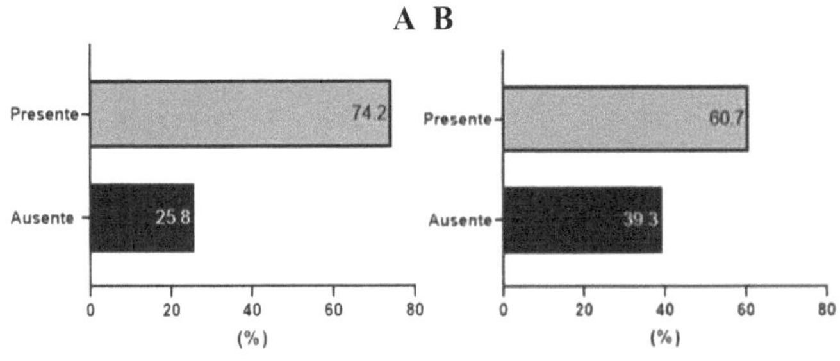

Source: Author

Regarding the drug information, it was observed that 39.3% (70) did not have the pharmaceutical form of the drug (graph 4B). It is notorious that the lack of information in a prescription hinders the patient's treatment, which can be life-threatening. Despite this, the lack of information in prescriptions is relatively frequent in the routines of health services (SILVERIO, 2010).In 56.2% (78) the absence of drug concentration was identified (graph 5A), a higher value found by Miranda et al., (2014) which was 3.17%. Regarding the posology (graph 5B), 69.7% (124) of the prescriptions presented complete posology, 30.3%(54) did not present the posology, similar results found by Lucas et al, (2012). The lack of posology in prescriptions leads to administration of lower or higher doses than indicated, inefficiency of treatment and even adverse reactions, drug interactions, intoxications, or death of the patient (GIMENES et al, 2010). It was observed that the percentage of data related to concentration, posology, lower when compared with previous studies of Silvério; Leite (2010) and Firmo et al. (2013), which detected respectively 91.1% for information present on the concentration of the drug, and 86.3% for information on posology. These data are relatively important for filling in prescriptions, as they facilitate the rational use of the drug, since the lack of information in the prescription makes the patient's treatment more difficult and life-threatening.

Graph 5- Distribution of prescriptions according to the presence of drug concentration (A) and dosage (B)

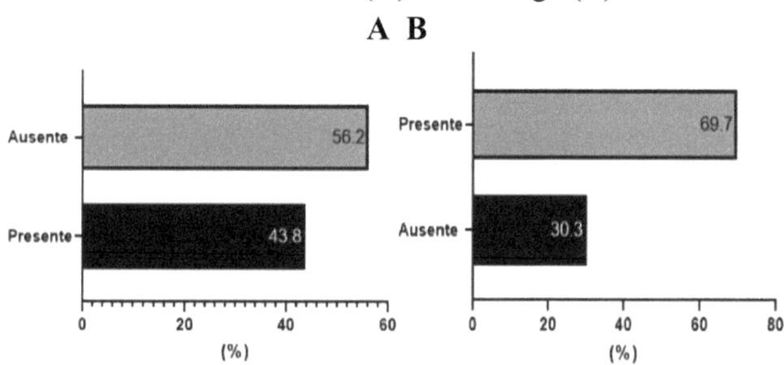

Source: Author

Graph 6 shows how long respondents have been using antidepressants. It can be observed that 60% have been taking them for a period of 1 to 5 years, 24% for more than 10 years, 8% between 5 and 10 years, and the other 8% for less than 1 year.

Graph 6 - Time of antidepressant use by the interviewees.

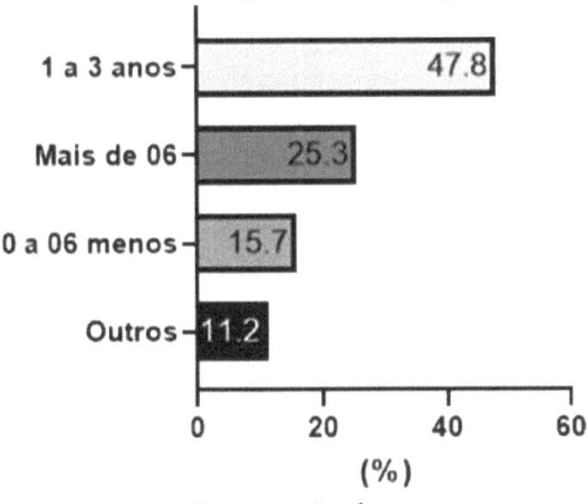

Source: Author

Regarding the time of treatment, it is observed that many patients have been using psychotropic drugs for years, i.e., most respondents are in treatment between 1 to 5 years. Silva et al. (2015) found in their data that respondents used psychotropic drugs for more than 3 years, in the same perception, Santos, Almeida and Estacio (2014) observed that many patients used these drugs for an average of 3 and 10 years. However, it is important that the communication between the pharmacist and the patient occurs at the time of dispensation, since it will create a bond between them, and thus contribute to the awareness of patients to appeal to the prescribing clinical professionals in order to monitor the evolution of treatment (SPAGNOL; IACOVSKI, 2010). According to Silva (2011), antidepressants are effective in the treatment of various psychiatric problems, however, they should not be prescribed chronically. The designated medication, dosage and treatment time should be appropriate to the patient's clinical needs, thus a frequent and careful medical analysis is essential. The prolonged use of antidepressants should not occur for more than three or four months, due to the loss of their sleep-inducing function and the possible side effects that their long-term use can bring (cognitive loss, decreased productivity, increased possibility of traffic accidents), in addition to the risks of developing tolerance and withdrawal symptoms, which could lead the patient, many times, to increase the dose to continue with the desired therapeutic effects (SIRDIFIELD et al., 2013; ALVARENGA et al., 2014).

CONCLUSION

An adequate prescription is an important step in the treatment process, because it directly influences the dispensing stage, where the pharmacist can participate in the care of drug users, interfering, mainly, in the use and adequate control, avoiding drug-related problems, which can lead to negative results to the medication. It is part of pharmaceutical care to sensitize patients to always seek medical intervention and follow-up in order to monitor the clinical evolution of the treatment, and when appropriate, to modify and adapt the therapy, considering the long-term effects of antidepressant use.

REFERENCES

ANTHIERENS, S., PASTEELS, I., HABRAKEN, H., STEINBERG, P., DECLERCQ, T.,CHRISTIAENS, T. Barriers to non-pharmacologic treatments for stress, anxiety, and insomnia: Family physicians' attitudes toward benzodiazepine prescribing. **Canadian Family Physicianv**. 56, no. 11, p. 398-406, 2010.

ALVARENGA, J. M. et al. Chronic use of benzodiazepines among older adults. **Public Health Journal**, 2014.

ANDRADE, J. M.; SOUA, F. A. F.; DUARTE, J. F.; LEITE, P. I. P.; CARVALHO, P. M. Et al. Evaluation of Adherence to Antidepressant Treatment in Patients of a Public Pharmacy in the Interior of Ceará. **Id On-line**. V.12, n.42, p.203-212. 2018.

AZEVEDO, L.S., PEREIRA, L.J., ZANGERÔNIMO, M.G., SOUSA, R.V., MURGAS, L.D.S., MARQUES, L.S., CASTELO, P.M., PEREIRA, C.V. Avaliação da adequação legal of prescriptions and prescription notifications of drugs subject to special control from the public and private sectors. **Revista Ciências Farmacêuticas Básica Aplicada**. v. 32, nº 3, p.401 - 417, 2011.

Brazil. Federal Council of Medicine. Resolution No. 1931 of September 17, 2009. Approves the Code of Medical Ethics. Diário Oficial da União 13 oct 2009; Section 1.

CANADIAN PHARMACISTS ASSOCIATION. **The Role of Pharmacists in Improving Community Mental Health,** vol. 4, no. 9. 2015.

EV, L. S.; GUIMARÃES, A. G.; CASTRO, V. S. Evaluation of prescriptions dispensed in a Primary Health Care Unit in the city of Ouro Preto, Minas Gerais, Brazil. Latin **American Journal of Pharmacy,** v. 27, n.4, p.543-547, 2008

FERRARI, C. K. B.; BRITO, L. F.; OLIVEIRA, C. C.; MORAES, E. V.; TOLEDO, O. R;

DAVID, F. L. Failures in the prescription and dispensation of psychotropic drugs: A Public Health Problem. **Journal of Basic Applied Pharmaceutical Sciences**. v. 34, n. 1, p.109-116, 2013

FERRARI, C.K.B., BRITO, L.F., OLIVEIRA, C.C., MORAES, E.V., TOLEDO, O.R.,

DAVID, F.L. Failures in Prescribing and Dispensing Psychotropic Drugs: A Public Health Problem. **Journal of Basic Applied Pharmaceutical Sciences**. v. 34, no. 1, p. 109-116, 2013.

FIRMO, W. C. A.; PAREDES, A. O.; CUNHA, C. L. F.; TORRES, A. G.; BUCCINI, D. F.

Analysis of psychotropic prescriptions from a commercial pharmacy in the municipality of Bacabal, Maranhão. v.4, n.1, p.10- 18, 2013.

FIRMO, W. C. A. PAREDES, A. O, CUNHA, C. L.F, TORRES, A. G, BUCCINI, D. F.

Analysis of psychotropic prescriptions from a commercial pharmacy in the municipality of Bacabal, Maranhão. **Journal of Management and Primary Health Care.** 4(1):10-18.2013

FIOCRUZ. Cases of Drug Poisoning by Federated Unit, 2017.

GIMENES, F. R. E, MOTA, M. L. S, TEIXEIRA, T. C. A, SILVA, A. E. B. C, OPITZ, S. P,

CASSIANI, S. H. B. Patient safety in drug therapy and the influence of the medical prescription on dose errors. **Revista Latino-Americana Enfermagem**. 2010; 18(6):1055 1061. DOI: 10.1590/S0104- 11692010000600003.

LUCAS, J. C. F.; OLIVEIRA, M. C.; FONSECA, M. H. G.; FRANÇA, D. S.; RABELO, J.

A. **Evaluation of the profile of medical prescriptions collected in a drugstore in Montes Claros - MG.** Motricidade. 2012; 8(Supl.2):187-196.

MARQUES L.A.M., et al. Pharmaceutical care to patients treated with antidepressants.

Revista de Calidad Asistencial, vol. 27, no. 1, pp. 55-64. 2012.

MIRANDA, J. S.; FONTES, B. M. L.; FRANCO, A. J. Identificação de Inconformidades nas Prescrições Médicas da Unidade Básica de Saúde Guiricema, MG. Annals. VI SIMPAC, V 6,N. 1.2014.Available at https:// acadêmico.univicosa.com.br/revista/index.php/RevistaSimpac/article/dowload/42

1/6 14. Accessed on 05 Nov. 2020.

OLIVEIRA, A. P; ÁVILA, T, S; SOUZA, M. A. N.; FARIA, W. J. J. Levantamento
epidemiological profile of users of tricyclic antidepressants in four drugstores in the city of Rubiataba -GO from 2009 to 2011. **Electronic journal of the college of Ceres.** V.1,n.1. 2012

OLIVEIRA, C. S, SANTOS, A. S, LEITE, I. C. G. Avaliação da qualidade das prescrições médicas da farmácia municipal de Catalão-Goiás. **Revista Médica Minas Gerais.** 2015; 25(4):556- 61.

WORLD HEALTH ORGANIZATION. **Mental disorders. Geneva,** April 2016.

PINHO, P. S; ARAÚJO, T. M. Association between domestic overload and common mental disorders in women. **Brazilian journal of epidemiology.** V.15, n.3, p.560-572. 2012.

ROCHA, B. S.; WERLANG, M. C. Psychopharmaceuticals in the Family Health Strategy: utilization profile, access and strategies for the promotion of rational use. **Revista Ciência e Saúde Coletiva,** v. 18, n. 11, p. 3291-3300, 2013.

ROCHA, B. S; WERLANG, M. C. Psychoactive drugs in the Family Health Strategy: profile of use, access and strategies for the promotion of rational use. **Ciência e saúde coletiva,** Rio de Janeiro, v. 18, n. 11, p. 3291-3300. 2013.

SANTOS, E. A; ALMEIDA, M. L. ESTÁCIO, S. C. S. A. Evaluation of the profile of psychotropic drug users in the municipalities of Tremembé and Pindamonhangaba. Monograph.

Library

Digital, Faculdade de Pindamonhangaba, São Paulo, 2014.

SILVÉRIO, M. S.; LEITE, I. C. G. Qualidade das prescrições em municípiode Minas Gerais: Uma
abordagem farmcoepidemiológica. **Revista da Associação Medica Brasileira.**2010; 56(6): 675-680.

SILVA, I. V. Adverse Effects of Antidepressant Use in the Elderly - Graduate Thesis. 2011.

SILVÉRIO, M. S, LEITE, I. C. G. Qualidade das prescrições em município de Minas Gerais: Uma abordagem farmacoepidemiológica. **Revista da Associação Medica Brasileira.** 56(6): 675- 680.2010.

SILVA, V. P.; BOTTI, N. C. L.; OLIVEIRA, V. C.; GUIMARÃES, E. A. A. Profile epidemiology of benzodiazepine users in primary health care. **Revista de Enfermagem do Centro Oeste Mineiro,** v. 5, n. 1, 2015.

SILVA, E. R. B, BANDEIRA, V. A. C, OLIVEIRA, K. R. Avaliação das prescrições dispensadas em uma farmácia comunitária no município de São Luiz Gonzaga-RS. **Revista de Ciências Farmacêuticas Básica e Aplicada**. 2012; 33(2):275-81.

SOUZA, A.R.L., OPALEYE, E.S., NOTO, A.R. Contexts and patterns of benzodiazepine misuse among women. **Science and Collective Health.** v. 18, no. 4, p.1131-1140, 2013.

SOARES, C. T. **Análise da prescrição de paroxetina em uma drogaria do município de ponte nova, minas gerais.** Annals VI SIMPAC - Volume 6 - n. 1 - Viçosa-MG - jan. - dec. 2014 - p. 101-106.

STOPA, S. R et al. Prevalence of self-reported depression in Brazil: results from the National Health Survey, 2013. **Brazilian Journal of Epidemiology.** V.18, n2. 2015.

SPAGNOL, W. P.; IACOVSKI, R. B. Uso de medicamentos psicotrópicos no programa saúde mental no município de água doce - SC. **Agora: Journal of Scientific Dissemination,** Mafra, v. 17, n. 1, 2010.

SIRDIFIELD, C. et al. General practitioners' experiences and perceptions of benzodiazepine prescribing: systematic review and meta-synthesis. **BMC Family Practice**. 2013

WAGNER, G. A., ANDRADE, A. G. Pharmacist professionals in the prevention of drug abuse: updating roles, and opportunities. **Brazilian Journal of Pharmaceutical Sciences.** São Paulo. v. 46, n. 1, p. 19 - 27, 2010.

PHARMACOTHERAPY PROFILE OF ELDERLY PATIENTS SEEN AT A PRIMARY PHARMACY.

[1] Pharmacy student, Faculdade de Integração do Sertão - FIS.

[2] PhD student at the Federal University of Pernambuco.

Amanda Natyele Magalhães de Lima [1]

José Israel Guerra Junior [2] Gabriela Cavalcante da Silva [3]

[3] Professor at the University of Pernambuco and at the Faculdade de Integração do Sertão.

SUMMARY

Introduction: Pharmacovigilance is defined as a set of activities aimed at identifying, evaluating, understanding, and preventing adverse effects. The elderly are a potential target of these adverse effects, since these patients do not have as much access to information as is necessary. They are also susceptible to polypharmacy, since they usually take more than 4 medications a day, thus causing possible drug interactions. **Objective: To** identify possible drug interactions caused by polypharmacy and classify them according to severity, promoting an analysis of the patient's pharmacotherapy, aiming at greater safety in their treatment together with the basic pharmacy. **Methodology:** This was a descriptive study, cross-sectional, with a quanti-qualitative approach. For this research, the prescriptions of 261 elderly patients seen at a basic pharmacy were used. **Results:** It was possible to observe 6.13% (16) cases of polypharmacy; 3.44% (7) interactions classified as mild, 78.32% (159) moderate and 18.22% (37) severe were identified. The most frequent mild interaction detected was Lithium Carbonate and Diazepam 42.85% (3). frequent was Fluoxetine and Clonazepam 13.20% (21), in the case of the severe, Amitriptyline and Fluoxetine 45.9% (17) was the most expressive. For prescription errors, three types were identified in prevalence, which were, Illegibility 55.30% (21), no date 44.70% (17), no stamp 18.40% (7). **Conclusion:** The need of a pharmacist for the correct evaluation of prescriptions is concluded, in order to guarantee a better pharmacotherapy to the patient.

Keywords: Polypharmacy. Pharmacotherapy. Drug Interactions

INTRODUCTION

According to the IBGE (2020), the average life span of a Brazilian citizen in 2019 is 76.6 years. This shows a progressive and rapid increase in the life expectancy of the older population. This fact is due to the improvement in the quality of life of citizens. Aging is a natural process of life, where physiological changes occur due to loss of homeostasis, which affects the immune system. Therefore, the effectiveness in protecting the human body against endogenous and exogenous agents is compromised, generating pathological conditions such as infectious, autoimmune, and neoplastic diseases (MACENA et al, 2018). The elderly class is the most practicing of polypharmacotherapy due to the high incidence of diseases acquired throughout life. The term polypharmacotherapy or polypharmacy suggests the use of several drugs simultaneously (BRAGA, 2019), and that in turn often results in drug interactions. These are classified into minor, moderate, and major. The minor one occurs where the type of interaction causes milder effects where they are not detected, in moderate degree the effects can clinically alter the patient's condition, and in greater degree the effects are severe and even lethal (SECOLI, 2010).It is estimated that 30% of hospital admissions by elderly patients are due to problems with medications, including toxic effects related to irrational use. This occurs due to the lack of monitoring or supervision of these patients, where they end up taking medications they don't need, confusing their medications, or even taking more than once a day of these drugs. The existence of polypharmacy exposes the elderly to a more difficult treatment, which requires increased attention, memory and organization about the schedule of drug administration, since the cognitive functions of the elderly are affected (ALMEIDA, 2017).According to the Federal Pharmacy Council (2020), between the years 2010 and 2017, 565,271 cases of intoxication were reported in Brazil. Among all these cases, 298,976 had medication as the toxic agent, which corresponds to 52.8% of all cases. Understanding the elderly population, taking into account its pharmacokinetic and pharmacodynamic aspects, is essential for strategies to be implemented, aiming to reduce the impact of health care spending, plan and propose strategies that provide improvements in health systems and better coverage to this age group (BALDONI et al, 2011). The use of drugs in health institutions has also caused an increase in prescription errors, thanks to the large number of drugs that make up the patient's history, leading to unwanted drug interactions. The errors in the administration of drugs are the result of several factors, among them can be mentioned, work overload of employees, physical and mental fatigue, lack of communication between professional and patient, and the similarity between many drugs (FRANTZ, 2012).Therefore, this work aimed to analyze the risks that the indiscriminate use of medicines brings to the elderly population, and consciously guide them about the safe practice of these drugs, verify the pharmacotherapy of the patient, looking for possible drug interactions and the incidence of polypharmacy in the city of Santa Cruz da Baixa Verde-PE.

METHODOLOGY

This was a descriptive, cross-sectional study, with a quanti-qualitative approach. The study was conducted in the municipality of Santa Cruz da Baixa Verde, located in the hinterland of Pernambuco, with a population of 12,708 inhabitants, according to the last Demographic Census of the IBGE, in the basic pharmacy of the municipality. For this research, the elderly patients were considered, who are seen and have their prescriptions filled in the basic pharmacy of the municipality, which has an average of 800 monthly visits considering the elderly population according to the number of management indicators. Based on the average monthly attendance, a total of 261 individuals and their prescriptions were considered for this research.The elderly were invited to participate in the research, with a brief explanation of the research objectives and further clarification. The copies were collected with prior consent and authorization of the patients, in question by signing the Informed Consent Form (ICF). Data collection was subsequently carried out after approval by the REC, and the data obtained were processed and analyzed according to the Drugs database, this tool was used to identify drug interactions and classify the clinical relevance of each interaction, observing and quantifying the patterns of prescription errors, and the incidence of polypharmacy in prescriptions. This research was duly approved by the Ethics and Research Committee of the Faculdade de Integração do Sertão, under opinion number 5,430,857 and CAAE number 57697122.3.0000.8267. Finally, the results obtained were categorized and plotted through graphs in the Gram Prisma program.

RESULTS AND DISCUSSION

The aging process consists of several organic modifications and consequently considerable physiological changes, such as, loss of functional tissue capacity, decrease in metabolic rate, increase in the amount of adipose tissue, substantial reduction of body fluids (MUNIZ et al. 2017).The sample of this study included data from 261 patients, using 95% reliability and 5% error. According to graph 1, 74.32% (194) were in the 60-70 age group; 20.68% (54) in the 71-80 age group; 4.21% (11) in the 81-90 age group; and 0.76% (2) over 100 years old.

Graph 1- Age range of the interview participants

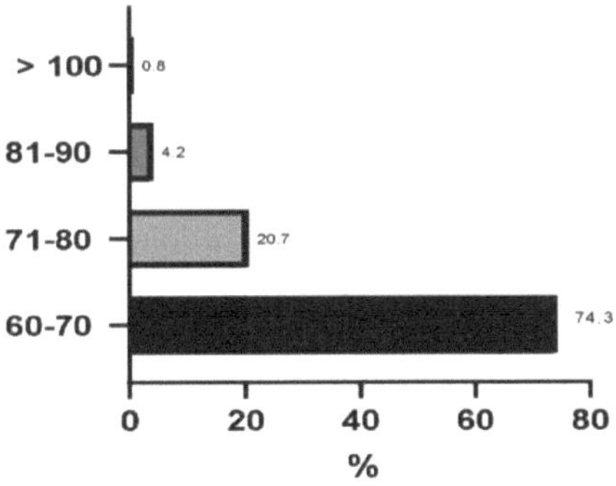

Source: Author

Polypharmacy is defined as the simultaneous use of four or more medications (ISMP, 2017). The increase of polypharmacy in the elderly class is determined by the predominance of chronic noncommunicable diseases that require the association of several drugs and by the way health care is carried out for the elderly, with different specialists who are unaware of the patient's drug history, and the increase in life expectancy and the consequent increase in multimorbidity (CARVALHO et al. 2012).This study showed that in the basic pharmacy of the city of Santa Cruz da Baixa Verde-PE, 6.13% (16) cases of polypharmacy were observed and collected. In a study conducted with the elderly in basic units of Belo Horizonte found the frequency of polypharmacy in 57.7% of patients (OLIVEIRA et al. 2021). Additionally, a study with conducted in the city of São Paulo, with home interviews conducted by previously trained professionals showed a percentage of 33% frequency of polypharmacy, being more frequent in women (36.6%) than in men (26.9%). The most prevalent age group was the elderly over 75 years old (41.3%) (ROMANO et al. 2018).Differing from this study, Rezende et al. (2021) based on home visits in rural and urban areas of Rio Branco with elderly people, evidenced 14.9% cases of polypharmacy, where the frequency was in white women. There was a higher prevalence of polypharmacy among the elderly who made a self-assessment of bad and very bad health, in those with signs and symptoms of depression, among the obese, hypertension, diabetes mellitus, insomnia, arthritis/arthrosis, osteoporosis, heart problems, dyslipidemia, and depression. Mascarelo et al. (2021) evidenced 29.3% of polypharmacy cases with the prevalence also in female patients in the public network in cities of Rio Grande do Sul. The main groups of drugs responsible for polypharmacy in the studied population were those with action on the digestive system and metabolism (95.4%), followed by those that act on the nervous system (88.5%).Drug interactions are defined as a phenomenon that occurs when the effects of a drug are modified by the anticipated or simultaneous administration of another drug (REBOLÇAS, 2016). In situations of polypharmacy, the possibility of drug interactions is increased. A total of 203 drug interactions could be detected in the evaluated prescriptions, thus there is an average of 0.77 frequency of interaction per prescription. Considering the cases of interaction, 3.44% (7) were identified as mild, 78.32% (159) as moderate and 18.22% (37) as severe, graph x.

Graph 2 - Classification of drug interactions

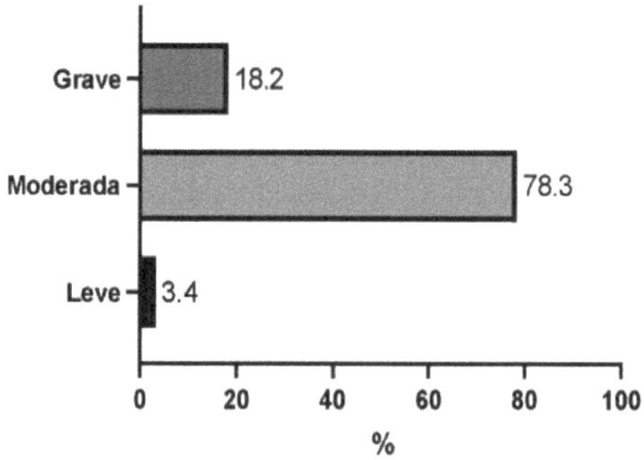

Source: Author

Drug interactions are defined as any harmful or undesirable, unintended response to a drug, which occurs at doses usually employed in man for prophylaxis, diagnosis, disease therapy or for the modification of physiological functions (RODRIGUES et al, 2016). Drug interactions are significant causes of hospital admissions and medical visits, accounting for up to 22.2% of adverse reactions leading to patient hospitalization (DECHANONT et al, 2014). For this reason, interactions should be observed in patients who use polydrug therapy. As illustrated in table 1, among the interactions identified as mild, 42.85% were (3) was between Lithium Carbonate/Diazepam and 28.57% (2) Fluoxetine/Valproic Acid. Lithium Carbonate associated with Diazepam may generate hypothermia, in addition to increasing the clinical effects of Diazepam, generating severe sedation, cardiovascular or respiratory depression. Fluoxetine can increase the bioavailability of Valproate by inhibiting its hepatic metabolism. Fluoxetine acts in the brain by raising levels of serotonin, the neurotransmitter responsible for regulating mood, concentration, among other functions (DRUGS.COM, 2022).

Table 1 - Most frequent drug interactions.

Serious Interactions		Frequency
Amitriptyline	Fluoxetine	17(45,94%)
Lithium Carbonate	Fluoxetine	4 (10,81%)
Haloperidol	Promethazine	4 (10,81%)

Moderate Interactions		
Fluoxetine	Clonazepam	21 (13,2%)
Amitriptyline	Clonazepam	18 (11,32%)
Biperidene	Clonazepam	8 (5,03%)

Mild Interactions		
Lithium Carbonate	Diazepam	3 (42,85%)
Fluoxetine	Valproic acid	2 (28,57%)
Carbamazepine	Phenobarbital	1 (14,28%)

Source: Author

In relation to the interactions classified as moderate, 13.20% (21) were related to the association of Fluoxetine/Clonazepam and 11.32% (18) were made up of the concomitant use of Amitriptyline/Clonazepam. Central nervous system and/or respiratory depressant effects may be intensified additively or synergistically in patients taking multiple drugs that cause these effects, especially in elderly or debilitated patients. Side effects such as dizziness, drowsiness, confusion, and difficulty concentrating may be more incisive in the association between clonazepam and fluoxetine. In the elderly it may affect thinking, judgment, and motor coordination (MEDSCAPE, 2022).Amitriptyline associated with clonazepam can cause dizziness, drowsiness, and breathing problems. Central nervous system and/or respiratory depressant effects may be additively or synergistically increased in patients taking clonazepam and tricyclic antidepressants (MEDSCAPE, 2022). Clonazepam belongs to a pharmacological class known as benzodiazepines, which have as their main properties, mild inhibition of Central Nervous System functions, thus allowing an anticonvulsant action, some sedation, muscle relaxation and tranquilizing effect (DOKKEDAL et al. 2019).In turn, among the serious interactions 45.9% (17) were in relation to Amitriptyline/Fluoxetine and 10.81% (4), was between Lithium Carbonate/Fluoxetine. Both amitriptyline and lithium carbonate associated with fluoxetine may increase the risk of serotoninergic syndrome, which may include symptoms such as hallucination, seizure, extreme changes in blood pressure, increased heart rate, fever, excessive sweating , chills or shaking, muscle spasm or stiffness, tremors stomach cramps, vomiting, and diarrhea. The same occurs for the use of lithium carbonate with fluoxetine (DRUGS, 2022). In the present study, 3 types of prescription errors were identified, such being illegibility 55.30% (21), followed by absence of date 44.70% (17), and absence of stamp 18.4% (7). A study conducted in a basic pharmacy in the Federal District in 2018, showed that of 1,063 prescriptions analyzed, only 64.5% (686) had completely legible spellings, presented some passage in which the reading was unrealizable (SANTOS et al, 2019).

Chart 3 - Most frequent prescription errors

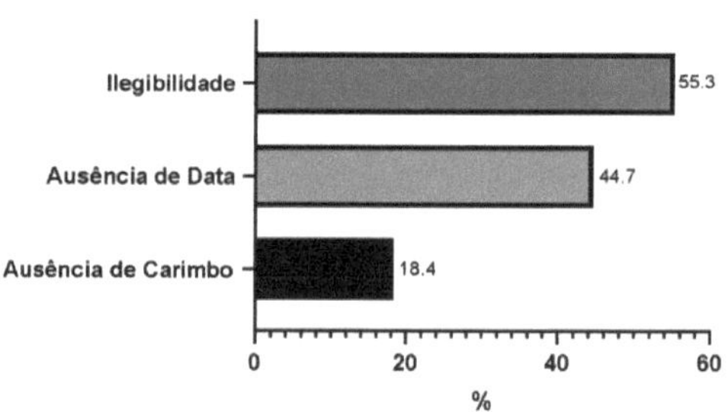

Source: Author

The lack of legibility of prescriptions leads to the possibility of confusion and makes it impossible for professionals to dispense medications correctly. According to Fernandes (2019), the implementation of electronic prescribing and the awareness of prescribers becomes fundamental for the reduction of medication errors and in turn, greater patient safety.

CONCLUSION

Considering the results obtained, it is concluded the need for the pharmaceutical professional in order to perform an evaluation of the prescriptions and thus ensure their validation, becoming this an essential work for patient safety. Prescription validation works as a barrier to minimize medication errors, identify drug interactions, and promote safety in pharmacotherapy. The pharmaceutical interventions performed are focused on avoiding medication-related problems before they generate negative medication outcomes.

REFERENCES

ALMEIDA, D.V.D. **Profile of the elderly patient admitted to a neurological Intensive Care Unit in a public hospital in the Federal District**. 2017. 107 f. Dissertation (Graduate Program in Nursing) - University of Brasília, Federal District, 2017.

BALDONI, A. L.; PEREIRA, L. R. O. Impacto do envelhecimento populacional brasileiro para o sistema de saúde sob a óptica da farmacoepidemiologia: uma revisão narrativa. **Journal of Basic Pharmaceutical Sciences** Apl., v.3, n.32, p. 313-21, 2011.

BRAGA, R. V. C; **Determinants of non-adherence to drug treatment of hypertensive users of a basic health unit.** 2019. 182 f. Dissertation (Professional Master in Family Health) - Federal University of Juiz de Fora, Juiz de Fora, 2019.

CARVALHO, M. F. C.; et al. Polypharmacy among the elderly in the municipality of São Paulo - SABE Study. **Revista Brasileira de Epidemiologia**, v.14, n.4, 2012.

CONSELHO FEDERAL DE FARMÁCIA. Perfil de intoxicação medicamentosa por auto-medicação no Brasil. Brasília: **Conselho Federal de Farmácia**, 2020 (Can be accessed at URL: https://www.cff.org.br/noticia.php?id=5849).

DECHANONT, S.; MAPHANTA, S.; BUTTHUM, B.; KONGKAEW, C.

Hospital admissions/visits associated with drug-drug interactions: a systematic review and meta-analysis. **Pharmacoepidemiol Drug Saf**. v. 23, n. 5, 2014.

DOKKEDAL-SILVA, V.; et al. Clonazepam: indications, side effects, and potential for nonmedical use. **Harvard review of psychiatry**, v. 27, n. 5, pp. 279-289, 2019.

DRUGS.COM. Drug Interaction Report. Available at: < https://www.drugs.com/drug_Interactions.php>. Accessed on: 20/05/2022.

FERNANDES, F. C. G. **Use of patient safety indicators in the analysis of the prescription and dispensing stages of medication**. 2019. 74 f. Dissertation (Master in Administration and Management of Pharmaceutical Care) - Universidade Federal Fliminense, Niterói, 2019.

FRANTZ, A. **Perception of nursing professionals about errors made in medication administration**. 2013. 30 f. Monografia (Trabalho de Conclusão de Curso)- Universidade Regional do Nordeste do Estado do Rio Grande do Sul, Ijuí, 2013.

IBGE - BRAZILIAN INSTITUTE OF GEOGRAPHY AND STATISTICS. **Characteristics ethnic-racial population:** classifications and identities. Rio de Janeiro: IBGE, 2020. Available at: https://agenciadenoticias.ibge.gov.br/agencia-sala-de-imprensa/2013-agencia-de-noticias/relea ses/29502-in-2019-life-expectancy-era-76-6-years. Accessed on: 20 May 2022.

ISMP. World Health Organization. Medication Without Harm - Global Patient Safety Challenge on Medication Safety. Geneva: World Health Organization, 2017. Available at: www.ismp-brasil.org/site/noticia/desprescricao-reduzindo-a-polifarmacia-e-prevenindo-erros- de-medicacao/.

MACENA, W. G.; HERMANO, L. O.; COSTA, T. C. Physiological changes due to aging. **Mosaicum Journal**, [S. l.], v. 15, n. 27, p. 223-238, 2018.

MASCARELO, A.; BORTOLUZZI, E. C.; HAHN, S. R.; ALVES, A. L. S.; DORING, M.; PORTELLA, M. R. Prevalence and factors associated with excessive polypharmacy in institutionalized elderly people in Southern Brazil. **Rev. bras. Geriatria e Gerontologia** v. 24 e. 2. Rio Grande do Sul. 2021.

MEDSCAPE. Drug interaction Checker. Available at: < http://reference.medscape.com/druginteractionchecker >. Accessed on: 20/05/2022.

MUNIZ, E. C. S.; et al. Analysis of the use of medications by elderly supplementary health plan users. **Revista Brasileira de Geriatria e Gerontologia**, v. 20, n. 3, p. 375- 387, 2017.

OLIVEIRA, P. C.; SILVEIRA, M. R.; CECCATO, M. G. B.; REIS, A. M. M.; PINTO, I. V.L.; REIS, E. A. Prevalence and Factors Associated with Polypharmacy in Elderly Patients Attended in Primary Health Care in Belo Horizonte-MG, Brazil. **Rev. Ciência Saúde coletiva** v.26 e.4. Belo Horizonte, Minas Gerais. 2021.

REBOUÇAS, W. L. S. **Analysis of drug-food interactions in the intensive care unit in a public hospital in the municipality of Mossoró/RN**. 2016. 64 f. Monograph (Course Completion Work) - Nova Esperança College of Nursing (FACENE), Mossoró, 2016.

REZENDE, G. R.; AMARAL, T. L. M.; AMARAL, C. A.; VASCONCELLOS, M. T. L;MONTEIRO, G. T. R. Prevalence and factors associated with polypharmacy in elderly residents in Rio Branco, Acre, Brazil: a population-based cross-sectional study, 2014. **Rev.Epidemiology and Health Services** v. 30 e. 2. 2021.

RODRIGUES, M. C. S; OLIVEIRA, C.; Drug interactions and adverse drug reactions in polypharmacy in the elderly: an integrative review. **Journal Latin American Nursing**, v. 24, 2016.

ROMANO-LIEBER, N. S.; et al. Elderly survival and exposure to polypharmacy in the municipality of São Paulo: SABE Study. **Revista Brasileira de Epidemiologia**, v. 21, 2019.

SANTOS, A. C. S.; et al. Prescription errors in a basic pharmacy in the Federal District. **Ciencia y enfermería**, v. 25, 2019.

SECOLI, S. R. Polifarmácia: interações e reações adversas no uso de medicamentos por idosos. **Revista Brasileira de Enfermagem,** v. 63, n. 1, p. 136-140, 2010.

BEHAVIOR OF PATIENTS SEEN BY A PHARMACOTHERAPY SUPPORT PROGRAM

¹ Pharmacy student, Faculdade de Integração do Sertão - FIS.
² PhD student at the Federal University of Pernambuco.
Stéphany Layane Freire Nogueira ¹ Rennan Luiz Leite Diniz ¹ José Israel Guerra Junior ² Gabriela Cavalcante da Silva ³
³ Professor at the University of Pernambuco and at the Faculdade de Integração do Sertão.

SUMMARY

Introdução: A Atenção Farmacêutica favorece a orientação e acompanhamento a terapia medicamentosa e sua relação direta paciente-farmacêutico, tendo em vista adesão a farmacoterapia e por sua vez, realiza-la de modo racional atinga resultados efetivos e favoráveis ao paciente. Objective: To analyze the behavior of patients assisted by a pharmacotherapy support program, in order to monitor their pharmacotherapy. Methodology: This was a descriptive, observational, cross-sectional, retrospective study with a quantitative and qualitative approach. Results: According to the data, 60% (63) of the patients who adhered to the support program were women; 64.8% (68) of the patients were responsive to follow-up; 37.2% (39) had comorbidities, the most frequent being Systemic Arterial Hypertension (SAH), Diabetes Mellitus (DM), Dyslipidemia (DL) and Heart Failure (HF).A percentage of 41% has the presence of possible drug interactions and classified according to their risk level, were 86.2% moderate, 7.3% severe and 6.4% mild. Conclusion: Taking into account the results obtained and based on a pharmacotherapy support program, new studies are still needed to promote the practice of pharmacotherapeutic monitoring and the importance of this conduct, as well as the implementation of programs like this in other drugstores and pharmacies.

Passwords: Pharmaceutical care. Clinical pharmacy. Pharmacotherapy.

INTRODUCTION

Pharmaceutical care (PA) was first defined in the 1990s by Hepler and Strand as "the responsible provision of drug treatment for the purpose of achieving concrete outcomes that improve patients' quality of life. This is performed by the pharmaceutical professional, ranging from drug therapy to decisions about the use of the given medication. It is considered the main pharmaceutical activity in clinical pharmacy, based on anamnesis, analysis, orientation, and follow-up processes (SANTOS, 2020).Thus, Pharmaceutical Care brings in itself the concept that the well being of the patient is the fundamental element of the actions of the pharmacist together with the multiprofessional team, in this case the physicians and other prescribers, to promote health. Belonging to pharmaceutical practice, developed in the composition of pharmaceutical assistance which includes attitudes, ethical values, behaviors, skills, commitments and co-responsibilities in the prevention, promotion and recovery of health in an integrated manner with the health team (BISSON, 2016). Through this practice, the professional can suggest measures that help in the treatment of the patient, also exercising the monitoring of the patient, and act in health education by performing preventive actions.

Pharmaceutical care can be performed through its clinical services, which are dispensing, pharmacotherapeutic monitoring, health education, pharmaceutical guidance, medication reconciliation, review of pharmacotherapy, among others (BARROS, 2019). Pharmacotherapy is composed of three main stages, being them: the initial pharmaceutical assessment (anamnesis), data interpretation, and orientation process. The pharmacist knows all aspects of the medications, offering the user greater access to information, who will start using these in a correct and safe way (BARBOSA et al, 2017). Besides this professional represents the last opportunity to identify, correct or reduce possible risks associated with therapy (CARVALHO et al, 2018). Pharmaceutical intervention is part of the process of pharmacotherapeutic monitoring and aims to solve and prevent negative outcomes arising from the use of medicines. In the research conducted by Araújo et al. (2017) data demonstrate that there is scientific evidence that pharmaceutical care improves clinical and economic outcomes. Pharmacotherapy can present problems in the need, effectiveness and safety of the drug, and through the detection of these problems, it is possible to determine what is interfering with therapeutic outcomes and the quality of life of the user (FREITAS, 2018). According to Nascimento et al. (2019), pharmacotherapy review enables pharmacists to apply their knowledge about health problems and medications, using studies through research, prevention and resolution of

Medication-Related Problems (DRP). Adherence to drug treatment occurs when the recommendations passed by the prescriber are properly followed by patients (CARVALHO A., 2020). Thus, a positive relationship between patients and health professionals, reflecting in lifestyle changes with healthy habits and thus collaborating in the pharmacological therapy (LEME et al., 2020).According to 2018 data from the Federal Pharmacy Council (CFF), there are more than 87,000 private pharmacies and drugstores in Brazil; this number makes the pharmacist the professional who is in a more strategic location, enabling wider access to the population. However, through bibliographic research it was noted the lack of articles that demonstrate the relevance of pharmacotherapy and in those found it is also perceived the lack of clinical pharmacy practice outside the hospital setting, a paradigm that in fact needs to be broken, especially because there is a need for pharmacotherapeutic treatment outside the hospital reality and pharmacies and drugstores have qualified pharmacists and are the most accessible health professional (OLIVERIA et al., 2017).Therefore, this study aimed to observe the reaction and behavior of the patients assisted by the treatment support program at Drogasil Serra Talhada 1, as well as their pharmacotherapy profile, and to assist them by providing support measures to make the therapy easier, more practical, and accessible to the patient's understanding.

MATERIALS AND METHODS

This was a descriptive, observational, cross-sectional, retrospective study with a quanti-qualitative approach, developed with the objective of demonstrating the profile of patient behavior, as well as the pharmacotherapeutic profile, based on a treatment support program offered by a private pharmacy. The research was carried out at DROGASIL SERRA TALHADA 1, a drugstore belonging to Raia Drogasil S/A, located in Serra Talhada in the state of Pernambuco. Based on the monthly attendance an average of 150 people adhere to the treatment support program. All the records of patients in the program for a period of three months were included in the research. After approval by the Research Ethics Committee of the Faculdade de Integração do Sertão -FIS, CAAE number: 57697022.1.0000.8267 and opinion number: 5.401.151, a data survey was carried out, which took place between the months of May and June 2022, of all the electronic medical records of the participating patients. The variables determined for this work were: age, gender, medications used, most prescribed therapeutic classes, probable comorbidities of the patients, incidence of polypharmacy, possible drug interactions, as well as their responsiveness to the program.The data were quantified and then formulated into tables and graphs. The possible drug interactions were evaluated from the Drugs Interactions Checker database, and were classified according to the level of risk.

RESULTS AND DISCUSSION

In this study, a total of 105 electronic medical records of patients seen by a pharmacotherapy support program were analyzed, the sample size was calculated considering 95% reliability and 5% margin of error, and the sample size was obtained through the monthly average of patients seen by the program in the drugstore in question, through the collection of retrospective data for the months of January to March 2022. Of the survey participants, 64.76% (68) were responsive to follow-up and a minority of 35.24% (37) were not responsive (Graph 1). (2020), which recognizes that there are still problems to be overcome for the improvement of pharmacotherapy monitoring in commercial pharmacies, among which stands out the fact that part of the population sees private pharmacies only as a commercial environment and not as a health environment, hindering the formation of bonds between pharmacist and patient and consequently limiting the possibility of pharmaceutical assistance, also correlating with the lack of programs similar to the analyzed that provide these behaviors.

Chart 1- Responsiveness of patients in the follow-up program.

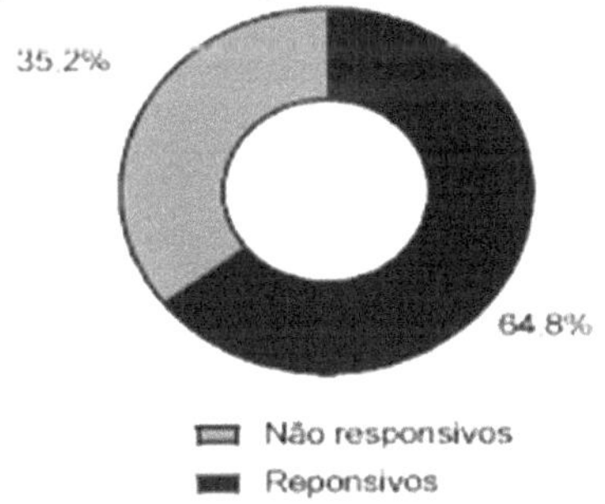

Source: Author

In graph 2 we have the classification in which 60% (63) of patients who joined the program are women and 40% (42) are men, thus, it is noted that gender can also be a crucial factor for adherence to drug therapy, strengthening what was exposed by Davis, et al. (2014) in a literature review, stating that in most studies the male gender is related to the worst percentage of adherence and there is better acceptance by women. However, Camuzi et al. (2021) reports that it is possible to find theses that point to both men and women, suggesting that the association of gender with adherence is not a determining factor.

Graph 2 - Classification by gender of the patients.

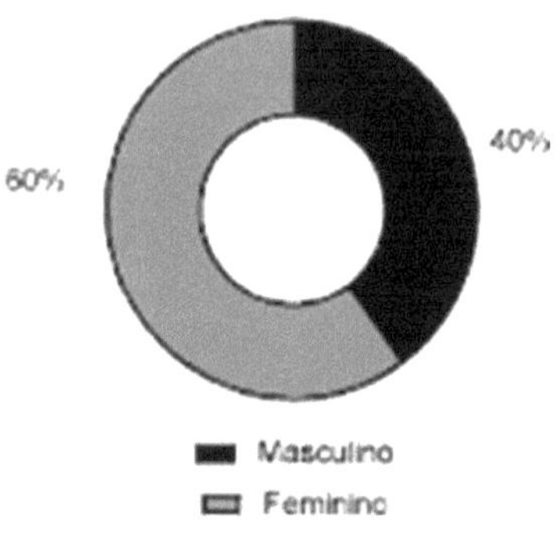

Source: Author

According to graph 3, 23.80% (25) of the participants correspond to the age group 31-40 years, 21.90% (23) between 21-30 years, 20% (21) within 41-50 years, 10.48% (11) 51-60 years old, 9.52% (10) from 61-70 years old, 5.71% (6) from 71-80 years old, and 8.60% (9) from 81-90 years old.

Graph 3 - Classification of patients by age group.

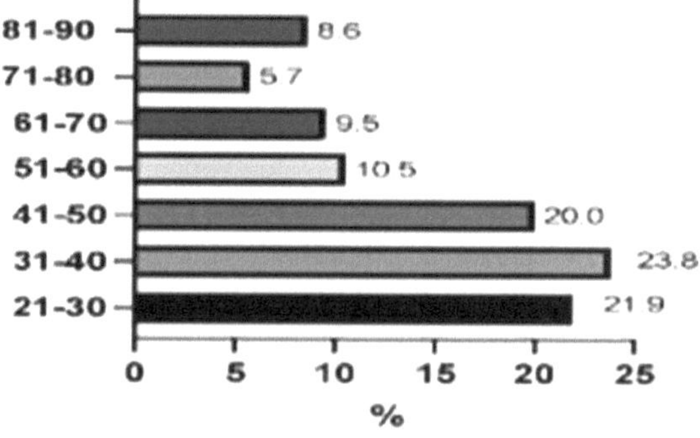

Source: Author

Souza and Soares (2018) say that because of the changes caused by aging, the elderly are more likely to present an evolution in pathologies and, in turn, increase drug consumption, consequently, the chances of administration errors and/or drug interactions. Bortolon et al. (2017) expose that the elderly have the need for continuous assistance because they present a higher rate of chronic diseases and occasionally need to be oriented in case of emergence of new health problems. In addition to being informed about the use of medications and their respective diseases.Caldas and Oliveira (2020) also reported that elderly patients undergoing treatment with various medications and continuously participating in pharmacotherapeutic follow-up experienced an important improvement of problems related to drug therapy and its repercussions, also favoring the aspect of self-care and a decrease in worries. They also showed, that through pharmacotherapy occurs the maintenance of quality of life and disease control, corroborating with Bortolon et al. (2017) who mentions that PA in the drugstore contributes significantly in care and improvement in quality of life.Among the participants 37.2% (39) had some comorbidity. 35,9% (14) have more than one comorbidity, while 64.10% (24) have only one, totaling 53 comorbidities. Of these, the most prevalent were respectively SAH (53.4%), DM (38.5%), HF (12.8%) and LD (30.8%) as described in graph 4, considering that some patients had more than one comorbidity. These results are compatible with the I Brazilian Registry of Heart Failure made by Albuquerque et al. (2015) with patients in hospitalizations in the public network in several regions of Brazil, which identified as the most prevalent comorbidities: hypertension, dyslipidemia, and diabetes, as well as Jorge et al. (2014), in a study of the prevalence of HF in the population in Niterói, found hypertension and diabetes as the most prevalent comorbidities.

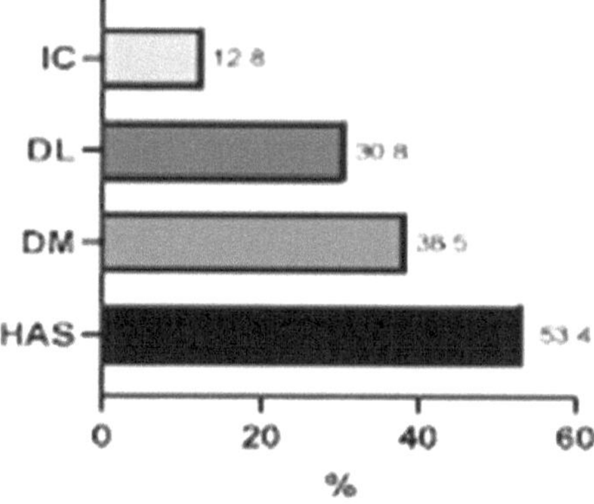

SAH: Hypertension; DM: Diabetes Mellitus; DL: Dyslipidemia; HF: Heart Failure.

Source: Author

As shown in graph 4, the comorbidity with the highest prevalence was SAH, which is a multifactorial clinical condition characterized by high and sustained levels of blood pressure (BP), considering BP values greater than or equal to 140/90mmHg (SOCIEDADE BRASILEIRA DE HIPERTENSÃO, 2017).Marques et al. (2021) emphasizes that the pharmacotherapy of SAH, the administration of medication is related to treatment outcomes and in some cases the use of polypharmacy is a desired condition to control and treat hypertension, reaffirming the need for guidelines for prevention and control of PRM. In sequence the DM with the morbidity of 28.30%, which is defined by multifactorial metabolic disorder associated with deficiency in the production and/or action of endogenous insulin, resulting in persistent hyperglycemia (FREITAS, et al. 2019).Barros et al. (2019) shows that in many cases monotherapy - treatment with a single medication - even at maximum doses cannot control glycemic indexes, thus having to add another medication, depending on each patient and their conditions. Thus, clinical pharmaceutical services, especially pharmacotherapeutic monitoring is effective and relevant in improving the quality of drug therapy and disease control (BARROS; SILVA; LEITE, 2020).The patients participating in the program used a total of 317 medications. Among the most used classes were antihypertensives 11.37% (36), followed by antibiotics 10.72% (34), 9.46% (30) NSAIDs, antidepressants with a percentage of 8.72 (27) and a smaller portion of hypoglycemic agents 5.99% (19).

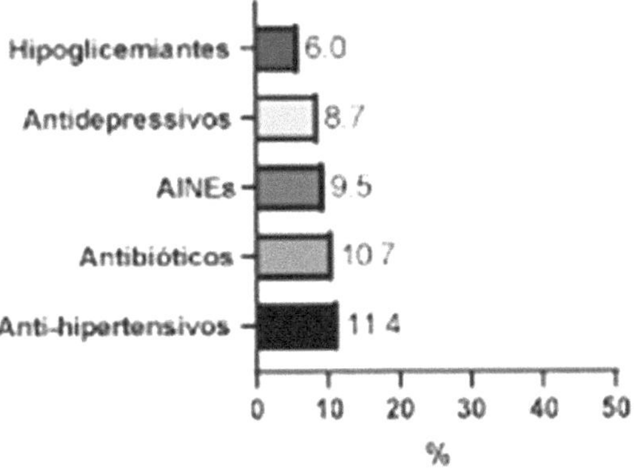

Source: Author

The prevalent use of antihypertensives is correlated to SAH being the most frequent comorbidity in the group studied, also linked to the treatment that does not respond satisfactorily to monotherapy requiring drug combinations in order to enhance the effectiveness of antihypertensives (MARQUES et al. 2021). As well as the association with other diseases and the emergency use of other drugs, thus making the use of more drugs.Veloso et al. (2019) argues that although the medication reconciliation is recommended and presents positive results, it generates an increase in the number of medications used, configuring polypharmacy and its inappropriate use can cause PRM, such as adverse effects, drug interactions, therapeutic ineffectiveness, and poor adherence to treatment. The common and simultaneous use of four or more medications (per prescription) is characterized by polypharmacy (ISMP, 2018). Reaffirming, Neto et al. (2021) argue that it can be one of the determining factors for the carelessness in taking medication schedules, besides the ingestion of several daily pills increasing the chances of drug interaction and therefore causing intoxication and compromising the patient's health. In the data analyzed, 31.43% (33) use polypharmacy (graph 6), and of these, 58% (19) are elderly.

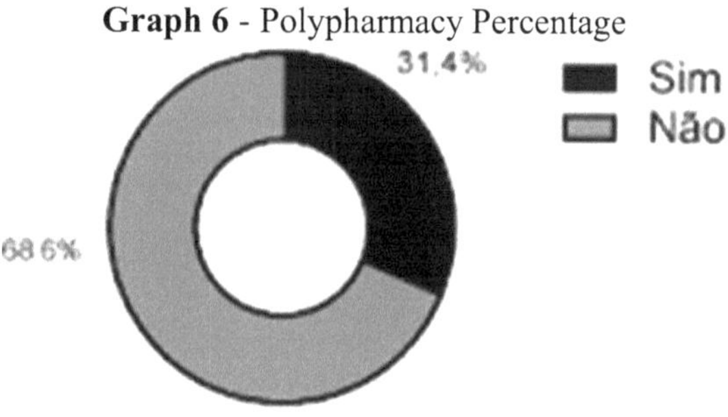

Source: Author

As for the frequency of Antibiotics and Over-the-Counter Drugs (OTCs) shown in chart 7, a 20% (21) percentage of patients used only OTCs, 11.4% (12) used antibiotics, and 15.2% (16) used both classes of drugs.

Graph 7 - Frequency of IPMs and Antibiotics

Source: Author

The National Health Surveillance Agency (ANVISA) defines PIMs as drugs that have approval by the health agency, being directed to the therapy of ailments considered as minor and that can be marketed without the need for prescription (ANVISA, 2016). Guimarães et al. (2021) cites in their studies that over-the-counter drugs require health authorization to be marketed in pharmacies and drugstores, and are used to treat self-limited problems without requiring a prescription for dispensing, given that they are safe and effective when used according to the guidelines described in the package inserts and labels.In the data analyzed, the frequency of use of PIMs, whether individualized or associated with the official prescription, is seen with a higher percentage; which is in accordance with the literature review made by D' Agostini (2018), which says that PIMs are the most consumed in Brazil and although it has variations it still points out the classes of analgesics, antipyretics, and anti-inflammatories and the drugs, dipyrone and paracetamol as the most used. Due to the easy access Pedott (2018), in a survey conducted with patients at a pharmacy in Erechim-RS, justifies that the need to get immediate relief associated with the difficulty of getting care in the Unified Health System or private, enhance the search for these drugs.However, Cruz Junior (2021) points out that the use of PIMs without the proper responsibility and the self-medication of these can lead to health risks such as aggravation of disorders, delay for proper diagnosis, risk of dependence, intoxications, allergic reactions, adverse effects, and drug interactions if the patient is already using others. Due to this, the pharmacist must offer to the patient the service of management of self-limited problems to their needs, prescribing and providing orientation regarding the use of PIMs and non-pharmacological measures, and if necessary refer the patient to another professional or health service (MIRANDA, et. al. 2021).In order to have control with dispensation and marketing of antimicrobials, ANVISA created the Resolution of the Collegiate Directorate - RDC No. 20 of 05 largest 2011 that provides for the control of medicines based on substances classified as antimicrobials, which regulates the dispensation in an attempt to properly follow the form of acquisition, dispensation and use of these, eradicating errors that contribute to the development of bacterial resistance (COSTA et al., 2019). Thus, the antibiotic being prescribed by a qualified professional, the pharmacist is responsible for the guidance and monitoring of this treatment, helping for greater safety and effectiveness of the patient and contributing to the reduction of bacterial resistance (ESTRELA, 2018).Silva et al. (2019) in a research on MI in prescriptions for the elderly in Minas Gerais, showed that among the drugs prescribed simultaneously with antibiotics, NSAIDs were more frequently prescribed, with similar results to the present study, due to the fact that they are drugs commonly used for the treatment of symptoms associated with infectious processes. Brito et. al (2016) highlighted in a study on the profile of the dispensation of antibiotics performed in Uruana - GO that the indiscriminate use of these drugs can be minimized as a result of pharmaceutical assistance, besides optimizing the antibiotic therapy, preventing and identifying PRM and thus guiding the patient to finish the therapy successfully, without interruptions, even after reduction of signs and symptoms.In the analyzed medical records, it was identified that 59% (62) have no incidence of Drug Interaction (MI) because they are medications with lower levels of interaction, or because the patients use fewer medications, while in the other 41% (43) a total of 109 possible interactions were found among the drugs used by them (Graph 8).

Graph 8 - Percentage of possible interactions.

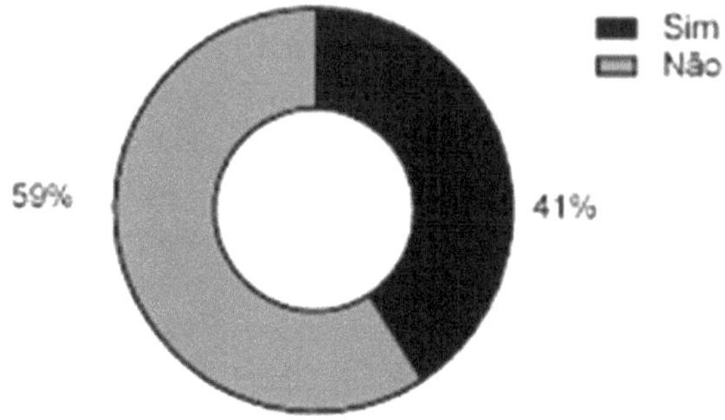

Source: Author

Drug interaction often happens due to the concomitant administration of drugs whose effects of the active ingredient are modified due to another. Some MI manifest potential can cause harm, and are responsible for the clinical worsening of the patient, increase in hospitalization time, on the other hand, others are mild and do not require special measures (CAVALCANTE et al., 2019). According to the database Drugs Interactions the more drugs an individual administers, the greater the chance of their drug interacting with another, and may decrease the effectiveness of their medications, and thus increase unexpected minor or serious side effects and even increase the blood level and possible toxicity of a particular drug.Most of the MI found were those classified as moderate with 86.24% (94), 7.34% (8) of severe level and 6.42% (7) mild, graph 9. In the research with the elderly in Minas Gerais conducted by Gotardelo et. al. (2014) shows the incidence of moderate interactions of 81.6%, 12.8% considered severe and 5.6% of light level, having the moderate interactions as the most frequent and the least the light interactions, which is relative to the data analyzed in the research in question. Additionally in the analysis of drug interactions in elderly patients in a pharmacy made by Cavalcante (2019) in Fortaleza - CE, also detected a higher prevalence of moderate MI with a percentage of 76.92%.

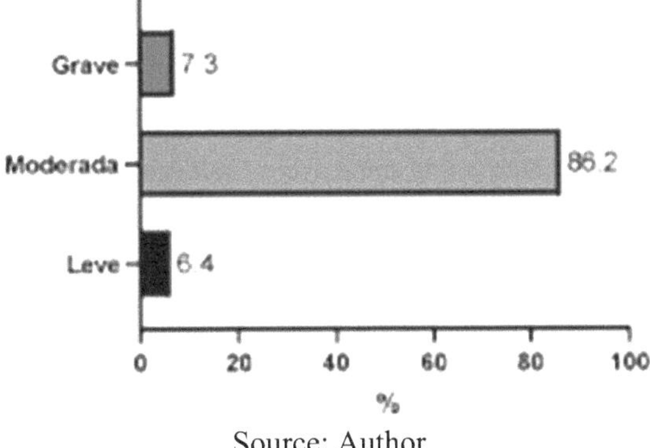

Source: Author

Potential Drug Interactions (PDIs) are classified according to severity as most severe when the interaction may be life-threatening and/or require medical intervention to prevent or lessen serious adverse effects; moderate, when the interaction may result in a marked patient health problem and/or requests a change in treatment; and minor when the interaction is limited clinical effects (MICROMEDEX, 2018).Of the most identified moderate MI, the use of antihypertensive diuretics with oral hypoglycemic agents stands out, being similar to studies developed with elderly patients with SAH and DM in Montes Claros - MG by Damasceno et. al (2019), which emphasized that the increased prevalence of chronic degenerative diseases diagnosed simultaneously, such as SAH and DM, has contributed to the incidence of drug interactions of clinical relevance, being possible to observe numerous harmful effects in patients under concomitant treatment of antihypertensive and oral hypoglycemic agents. As the interactions found in the present study between Hydrochlorothiazide with Metformin Hydrochloride where possible renal failure and dehydration induced by the use of diuretics may increase the risk of lactic acidosis in patients taking metformin concomitantly in addition, thiazides and other diuretics may interfere with glucose control, causing hyperglycemia, i.e. Hydrochlorothiazide decreases the antihyperglycemic effect of metformin, corroborating with Lima et al. (2015) who studied drug interactions in the treatment of type 2 diabetics. Regarding severe MI, the most common was Anlodipine with Simvastatin which can cause increased bioavailability of Simvastatin and increased risk of myopathy, including rhabdomyolysis, which can cause kidney damage and lead to death besides increasing the risk of side effects such as liver problems (DRUGS, 2022). Similar results were also obtained by Damasceno et al. (2019)

in a study conducted in Montes Claros.Thus, the dosage of simvastatin should not exceed 20 mg per day when used simultaneously with anlodipine, making it necessary to carefully consider this combination, along with multidisciplinary monitoring by a physician and pharmacist to the user. As for mild drug interactions, these do not usually cause harm or require any change in drug therapy. Levothyroxine and simvastatin were highlighted, IM which according to Drugs, simvastatin reduces or inhibits the pharmacological effects of thyroid hormone, with the mechanism of action as yet unknown. Especially, in isolated cases patients stabilized on levothyroxine trigger hypothyroidism symptoms and/or elevated thyroid stimulating hormone (TSH) levels after combination with simvastatin, in which case thyroid hormone dosage may need to be adjusted.The Rational Use of Medicines, which refers to the circumstance in which the patient uses the medicine appropriately to their clinical condition, in doses that are compatible with their needs, for an appropriate period of time, also considering the cost-benefit. In this way, the irrational use occurs when the patient does not know or ignores any of these steps, which can generate negative consequences on the health of the general population, but especially the elderly, highlighting that most of these adverse events have an avoidable nature and identifiable by health professionals (LIMA, et al. 2017).

CONCLUSION

Taking into consideration the results obtained in this study, one can notice the relevance of the pharmacotherapeutic treatment support, adequately and excellently performed by a pharmaceutical professional, through conducts that promote clinical activities such as pharmaceutical interventions that can detect potential drug interactions and other drug-related problems through initial analysis, prescription validation, thus avoiding damage to the patient's health and obtaining effective and satisfactory results in drug therapy. However, studies that show pharmacotherapy outside the hospital environment are still scarce, making it necessary to develop new studies that promote the practice of pharmacotherapeutic monitoring and its importance in community pharmacies, in the same way that it requires the implementation of support programs such as the one in the drugstore in question.

REFERENCES

ALBUQUERQUE, Denilson Campos et al. **I Registro Brasileiro de Insuficiência Cardíaca - Aspectos Clínicos, Qualidade da Assistência e Resultados da Internação.** Arq Bras Cardiol 2015,104(6):433-442.

ARAÚJO, Elaine de Oliveira; et al. Pharmaceutical interventions in an intensive care unit of a university hospital. **Brazilian Journal of Hospital Pharmacy and Health Services.** 08. 10.30968/rbfhss.2017.083.005.

BARROS, D. S. L.; SILVA, D. L. M.; LEITE, S. N. CLINICAL PHARMACEUTICAL
SERVICES IN BRAZIL'S PRIMARY HEALTH CARE. **Work, Education and Health**, v. 18, n. 1, 2020. Accessed on: 21 Feb. 2023

BARBOSA, M.; NERICOS. B. Pharmaceutical care as a promoter of the rational use of medicines. **Rev. unin revi**, v.30, n2. Jan, 2017.

BISSON, Marcelo. **Farmácia clínica & Atenção farmacêutica**. 3. ed. Barueri, SP: Editora Manole, 2016.

BORTOLON; et al. **Self-medication versus pharmaceutical indication: the pharmacy professional in primary health care for the elderly.** APS Journal, v.10, n.2, 2017, p. 200-209.

COSTA, J. M. DA et al. Restrictive measure for the commercialization of antimicrobials in Brazil: results achieved. **Revista de Saúde Pública**, v. 53, p. 68, 7 fev. 2019. Accessed on: 21 Feb. 2023.

BRITO, Adriane Ferreira; et al. **Profile of the dispensation of antibiotics in drugstores in the city of Uruana-GO. Revista Eletrônica da Faculdade de Ceres**, v. 5, n. 2, 2016.

CALDAS, Ana Lúcia Leitão; et al. Perceptions of elderly pharmacist services on polymedication. **Revista Brasileira de Enfermagem**, 73(5), pp. 1-8, DOI: 10.1590/0034-7167-2019-0305. 2020.
CAMUZI, Ranieri Carvalho; et al. Adesão farmacoterapêutica em insuficiência cardíaca: estudo exploratório num centro especializado fluminense. **Brazilian Journal of Health Review**, Curitiba, v.4, n.6, p. 26064-26082 nov./dec. 2021n

CARVALHO, Alanna Thereza De Farias; et al. **Adherence to pharmacological and non-pharmacological treatment in the elderly with hypertension: a literature review.** Annals of the

VII CIEH. Campina Grande: Realize Editora, 2020.

CARVALHO, Domingos Sávio de; et al. **Pharmacotherapy follow-up in respiratory intensive care unit: description of analysis and results.** Einstein (São Paulo). v,16, n2, 2018.

CARVALHO, Silas Santos; OLIVEIRA, Bruno Rodrigues de. The difficult adherence of hypertensive patients to treatment: Literature review. **Saúde Em Revista,** v. 18, n. 50, p. 53-64, 2020.

CAVALCANTE, Maria Lígia Silva Nunes et al. **Drug safety in institutionalized elderly: potential interactions.** Escola Anna Nery, v. 24, n. 1, 2019

CRUZ JUNIOR, Alex Fabiano da. **Self-medication of Over-the-Counter Drugs (OTC).** 2021.

CRUZ, Lais Helena de Lima et al. **Factors related to non-adherence to medication in the treatment of hypertension: an integrative review**. Course completion paper (Graduação) - Bacharelado em Enfermagem. Universidade Federal de Campina Grande - UFCG, Campina Grande-PB, 2017.

DA COSTA, Anderson Luiz Pena; JUNIOR, Antonio Carlos Souza Silva. **Bacterial resistance to antibiotics and Public Health: a brief literature review.** Estação Científica (UNIFAP), v. 7, n. 2, p. 45-57, 2017.

D'AGOSTINI, Charliane Patricio. **Pharmaceutical care in Brazil: a literature review.** 2018.

DAMASCENO, Eurislene Moreira Antunes; et al. Drug Interaction between Antidiabetics and Antihypertensives in the Elderly. **Multitexto Journal,** v. 7, n. 2, 2019.
DAVIS E.M; et al. The role of the pharmacist in predicting and improving medication adherence in patients with heart failure. **J Manag Care Spec Pharm,** v. 20, n. 7, p. 741-55, Jul 2014.

MIRANDA FILHO, Jorge Paulo; et al. **Pharmaceutical care and over-the-counter drugs: integrative literature review.** ARCHIVES OF HEALTH INVESTIGATION, v. 10, n. 1, p. 153-162, 2021.

BRAZILIAN HYPERTENSION SOCIETY GUIDELINES: 2016-2017. **Sociedade Brasileira de Hipertensão**; [organization José Egídio Paulo de Oliveira, Sérgio Vencio]. - São Paulo: Editora Clannad, 2017.

DRUGS. Drugs interactions Checker. **Drugs.com**. Last updated: 16-05-2022. Available at: https://www.drugs.com/drug_interactions.html. Accessed May 20, 2022.

Estrela, T. S. **Antimicrobial resistance: multilateral approach and Brazilian response. Advisor for International Health Affairs (MS).** v. 20, p. 1998-2018, 2018.

FREITAS, Daniele; et al. Negative outcomes associated with medication in hypertensive and diabetic elderly. **Journal Health NPEPS**, Mato Grosso, v.4, n.2, p. 118-131, Dec. 2019.

FREITAS, Jacqueline Gleice Aparecida; et al. Adherence to logical treatment in hypertensive elderly: an integrative review of the literature. **Rev Soc Bras Clin Med**, v. 13, n. 1,pp. 75-84, 2015

GOTARDELO, Daniel Rian; et al. Prevalence and factors associated with potential drug interactions among the elderly in a population-based study. **Rev Bras Med Fam Comunidade**. Rio de Janiero; v. 9, n. 31, p. 111-118, 2014.

GUIMARÃES, Pedro Henrique Damascena; et al. Pharmaceutical care and the use of Over-the-Counter Drugs (OTCs). **Research, Society and Development,** v. 10,n. 12, pp. e485101220405-e485101220405, 2021.
ISMP.World Health Organization Medication Without Harm - Global Patient Safety Challengeon Medication Safety. **Geneva: World Health Organization,** 2018. Available at:
www.ismp-brasil.org/site/noticia/desprescricao-reduzindo-a-polifarmacia-e-prevenindo-erro s-de-medication/.
JORGE, A. J. L. **Prevalência de função cardíaca na assistência pelo Programa Médico de Família de Niterói - RJ [thesis].** Niterói: Faculdade de Medicina - Universidade Federal Fluminense, 2014.

LEME, Camile de Mattos; et al. Predictors factors of non-adherence to antihypertensive drug treatment: integrative review. **Revista Saúde em Foco -** Edição nº 12, pág 324-331, 2020.

LIMA, R. F.; et al. Potential drug interactions in type 2 diabetics participating in a health education program. **Infarma - Pharmaceutical Sciences**, v. 27, n. 3, p. 160-167, 2015.

MARQUES, F. C. U; et al. Avaliação da prevalência da dispensação de antimicrobianos na farmácia pública do município de Cruz Alta - RS. **Revista eletrônica de farmácia,** v. 12, n. 2, p. 01-15, 2015.

MARQUES. J. de M. S.; BAIENSE, A. S. R. CONSULTÓRIO FARMACÊUTICO EM
DROGARIA. **Ibero-American Journal of Humanities, Sciences and Education**, v. 7, n. 10, p. 1627-1641, 2021.

MICROMEDEX® Solutions [Internet]. Accessed: 2018 October 20. Available from:
http://www.micromedexsolutionscom.ez127.periodicos.capes.gov.br/micromedex2/librarian.

NASCIMENTO, Mateus Oliveira; et al. Impact of pharmacotherapy complexity on biochemical and blood pressure parameters in diabetes mellitus. **Scientia Medica**, v. 29, p. e33175, 2019.

NETO, José Antônio Chehuen; et al. Prevalence of non-adherence to medication antihypertensive therapy in a sample from the city of Juiz de Fora-MG. **HU Magazine**, v. 47, p.1-9,2021.

OLIVEIRA, Naira Villas Boas Vidal de et al. Professional performance of pharmacists in Brazil: sociodemographic profile and work dynamics in private pharmacies and drugstores. **Saúde Sociedade.** v. 26, p. 1105-1121, São Paulo, 2017.

PEDOTT, Leticia. **Analysis of the use of over-the-counter medications by patients of a pharmacy in the city of Erechim-RS.** 2018.

SANTANA, Danubia Pereira Honório; et al. **A Importância da Atenção Farmacêutica na Prevenção de Problemas de Saúde. Revista de Iniciação Científica e Extensão**, [S. l.], v.2, n. Esp.1, p. 59-60, 2019.

SANTOS, B. V. A **prática do Cuidado Farmacêutico como ferramenta de redução de gastos do SUS e melhoria da qualidade de vida do indivíduo.** 36p. Course Conclusion Paper in Pharmacy-Biochemistry - Faculty of Pharmaceutical Sciences - University of São Paulo, São Paulo, 2020.

SILVA, Maria Eduarda de Freitas et al. **Influence of advertising on the use of over-the-counter medications by the elderly: A review.** 2019

SILVA, Larissa Santos; et al. Drug interaction analysis of prescriptions containing antimicrobials from a private drugstore in Minas Gerais. **Journal of Management & Primary Health Care**, ISSN 2179-6750, v. 10, 2019.

SOUZA, Robson Dias de; SOARES, Denise Josino. **Pharmaceutical care in the health of the elderly.** Coursework (Specialization in Family Health) - Institute of Health Sciences, University of International Integration of Afro-Brazilian Lusophony, São Francisco do Conde, 2018.

VELOSO, R. C; et al. Factors associated with drug interactions in elderly patients admitted to a high-complexity hospital. **Cien Saude Colet**. v. 24, n. 1, p. 17-26, Jan. 2019.

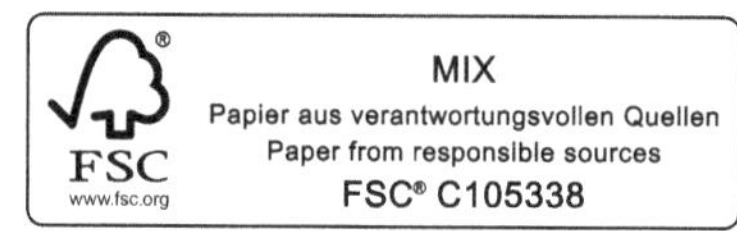

Printed by Books on Demand GmbH, Norderstedt / Germany